Paleobetic Diet

Defeat Diabetes and Prediabetes
With Paleolithic Eating

Visit us on the Internet
for updated information:

http://paleobeticdiet.com

Also by Steve Parker, M.D.:

The Advanced Mediterranean Diet:
Lose Weight, Feel Better, Live Longer (2nd Ed.)

Conquer Diabetes and Prediabetes:
The Low-Carb Mediterranean Diet

KMD: Ketogenic Mediterranean Diet

Paleobetic Diet

Defeat Diabetes and Prediabetes
With Paleolithic Eating

Steve Parker, M.D.
Sunny Parker

pxHealth

First edition published 2015
ISBN 978-0-9894775-9-8
Library of Congress Control Number: 2014908839

Published by pxHealth
PO Box 27276
Scottsdale, Arizona 85255 USA
Phone: (480) 695-3192
Web: http://pxHealth.com

Publisher's Cataloging-in-Publication data

Parker, Steve (Steven Paul).
    Paleobetic Diet : Defeat Diabetes and Prediabetes With
Paleolithic Eating / Steve Parker, M.D., Sunny Parker.
    pages cm.
    ISBN 978-0-9894775-9-8
    Includes bibliographical references and index.

1. Diabetes --Diet therapy. 2. Prediabetic state --Patients
--Diet therapy. 3. Diabetes--Nutritional aspects. 4. Prehis-
toric peoples --Food. 5. Nutrition. I. Parker, Sunny. II.
Title.

RC662 .P37 2015
616.4/620654 --dc23   2014908839

CONTENTS

Appendix

Dedicated to Paleolithic diet pioneers:

Walter L. Voegtlin, S. Boyd Eaton, Melvin Konner, Marjorie Shostak, Arthur De Vany, Ray Audette, Loren Cordain, Kerin O'Dea, and Keith Thomas

Disclaimer

The ideas and suggestions in this book are provided as general educational information only and should not be construed as medical advice or care. All matters regarding your health require supervision by a personal physician or other appropriate health professional familiar with your current health status. Always consult your personal physician before making any dietary or exercise changes. The publisher and authors disclaim any liabilities or warranties of any kind arising directly or indirectly from the use of the Paleobetic Diet. If any problems develop, always consult your personal physician. Only your personal physician can provide you medical advice

1
Introduction

THE PREMISE

If you found an injured bird in your backyard and wanted to nurse it back to health, how would you go about it? You'd have to do some research to improve your odds of success. First, what kind of bird is it? A sparrow? Robin? Hummingbird? Bluebird? An Owl?

You figure most birds are going to need some water. That's easy. (How does a hummingbird drink, anyhow?)

But what does that bird eat? Some eat plants only, and only certain parts of particular plants. Others eat insects or worms, and, then again, only specific insects and worms. Yet others, such as the owl, may only eat small mammals, lizards, and snakes. This is why identification of the bird species is so important. When you know that, you can google it to find out what to feed it. The owl will perish if you feed it birdseed; the sparrow will starve to death if all you offer to eat is mice.

Each bird species has evolved over hundreds of thousands of years to eat only certain foods. Nature provides the bird kingdom with seeds, berries, and other plant parts, insects, worms, and other animals to eat. But the skills and capacity to hunt, gather, and digest those foods are very specialized. It's a rare bird species that can use all those types of food to stay alive and, ultimately, to reproduce.

So, to be successful with your bird's rehabilitation, you need to find out what it needs to thrive. The same logic applies whether you're caring for a frog, snake, fish, bunny, or lizard. All these species are adapted to thrive on a particular diet and set of environmental circumstances such as temperature, light, even altitude.

In a nutshell, that's the rationale for the Paleolithic diet. The human animal over the last two hundred thousand years has adapted to eating certain foods and not others. Our non-human ancestors evolved for two million years before that. Most of the foods we eat today didn't even exist 10,000 years ago. Could our health improve if we returned to our ancestral diet? Will our original diet rehabilitate us? That's the premise, and the promise, of the Paleolithic diet.

HISTORY OF THE "MODERN" PALEOLITHIC DIET MOVEMENT

Charles Darwin is the father of evolutionary theory, as outlined in his 1859 book, *On the Origin of Species*. You don't have to believe in evolutionary theory if you don't want to. I know fundamentalist Christians who reject evolutionary theory and believe the Earth and all living species were formed by God just 6,000 years ago. Maybe they're right. In either case, just think of the thought experiment above, about feeding an injured bird found in your backyard. All animals, and *we are animals*, need a certain diet to survive and thrive.

You may have heard of the Paleolithic diet only a couple years ago. But it's been under consideration by serious thinkers for at least the last 40 years. Here's a timeline for the modern Paleolithic diet movement, focusing on publications. It's certainly not comprehensive, but probably more than enough to bore you:

1939 - *Nutrition and Physical Degeneration* by Weston A. Price's is published. Not specifically related to the Paleolithic era, but it did convincingly make the point that many diseases of modern civilization may be caused by modern diets of non-indigenous over-processed foods.

1952 - *Primitive Man and His Food* by Arnold Paul De Vries is published.

1973 - Stephen Boyden's article "Evolution and Health" is published in *The Ecologist*.

1975 - *The Stone Age Diet: Based On In-Depth Studies of Human Ecology and the Diet of Man* is published by Walter L. Voegtlin, M.D.

1985 - "Paleolithic Nutrition. A consideration of its nature and current implications" by S. Boyd Eaton and Melvin Konner in the *New England Journal of Medicine*.

11

1987 - *Stone Age Diet* by Leon Chaitow (London: Optima).

1988 - *The Paleolithic Prescription: A Program of Diet and Exercise and a Design for Living* by S. Boyd Eaton, Marjorie Shostak, and Melvin Konner.

1997 - Paleodiet.com established by Don Wiss in January.

1997 - The Paleodiet (sic) listserv established by Dean Esmay and Don Wiss in March.

1997 - The Evolutionary Fitness online discussion list is created in April. Art De Vany is its anchor and Tamir Katz is a regular participant.

1997 - Jack Challem published the article "Paleolithic Nutrition: Your Future Is In Your Dietary Past" in April.

1999 - *Neanderthin* by Ray Audette is published.

2001 - Evfit.com established by Keith Thomas in November ("Health and Fitness in an Evolutionary Context").

2001 - *The Paleo Diet* by Loren Cordain, Ph.D., is published in December.

2001 - Wikipedia's page on Palaeolithic (sic) diet is created in April.

2005 - Art De Vany's first paleo blog.

2006 - *Exuberant Animal* by Frank Forencich is published.

2008 - Art De Vany's Las Vegas seminar.

2009 - *The Primal Blueprint* by Mark Sisson is published.

2009 - Art De Vany announces "The New Evolution Diet."

2010 - *The New York Times* features the paleo lifestyle in its fashion pages on January 8.

2010 - *McLean's* (Canada) publishes a general audience review of the paleo movement February 26.

2010 - *Food and Western Disease* by Staffan Lindeberg, M.D., Ph.D., is published in February.

2010 - Paleolithic lifestyle page is created on Wikipedia in March.

2010 - Emily Deans, M.D., establishes the Evolutionary Psychiatry blog in June.

2010 - *The Paleo Solution: The Original Human Diet* by Robb Wolf is published in September.

2011 - *The New Evolution Diet* by Art De Vany is published in December.

Contributors to this timeline include Keith Thomas, Paul Jaminet, Don Wiss, and Ray Audette. Any errors are mine.

ORIGINS OF THE PALEOBETIC DIET

In 2011, my patients with diabetes began asking me if the Paleolithic diet would help with management of their diabetes. I didn't know. I didn't know much about the Paleolithic diet, period. So I started looking into the medical literature on health effects of the diet. My inquiry concentrated on:

- What is the Paleolithic diet?
- Is it nutritionally sound?
- What are its effects on people with diabetes, particularly the effects on blood sugar levels?

I've spent much less time on evolutionary theory, anthropology, paleoanthropology, archeology, and paleobotany.

Thus far, there aren't many scientific studies of the health effects of the Paleolithic diet. But there are some, involving both the general population and diabetics. I've also been influenced by folks with diabetes who took the plunge and tried the Paleolithic diet, many of them without the blessings of their ignorant healthcare professionals. (Ignorant simply means lacking knowledge of the Paleolithic diet.) These diabetics wouldn't have made the lifestyle change if the standard treatment approaches had been working for them. All this evidence led me to the Paleobetic Diet.

SCOPE OF THE PROBLEM

Diabetes is the most important public health problem in the U.S. and most of the developed world. Researchers affiliated with the U.S. Centers for Disease Control predict that four of every ten Americans will develop diabetes, mostly type 2 which accounts for 90 to 95% of adult cases.

Type 2 is less serious than type 1 diabetes.

Type 1 diabetics have an immune system abnormality that destroys the pancreas's ability to make insulin. Type 1's will not last long without insulin injections. On the other hand, many type 2 diabetics live well without insulin shots. Of U.S. adults with diabetes, only 5% have type 1. For unknown reasons, the prevalence of type 1 diabetes in Americans under 20 rose by 23% between 2001 and 2009.

"Prediabetes" is what you'd expect: a precursor that may become full-blown type 2 diabetes over time. Blood sugar levels are above average, but not yet into the diabetic range. One in four people with prediabetes develops type 2 diabetes over the course of three to five years. Prediabetes is over twice as common as type 2 diabetes.

The rise of diabetes parallels the increase in overweight and obesity, which in turn mirrors the prominence of highly-refined sugars and starches throughout our food supply. These trends are intimately related. Dr. Richard K. Bernstein, notable diabetologist, wrote that, "Americans are fat largely because of sugar, starches, and other high-carbohydrate foods." Increasing obesity rates are only partly to blame for diabetes. Dr. Robert Lustig thinks sugar consumption is a major culprit, regardless of body weight and activity levels. Public health authorities 40 years ago convinced us to cut down our fat consumption in a mistaken effort to help our hearts. We replaced fats with body-fattening carbohydrates that test the limits of our pancreas to handle them. Diabetics and prediabetics fail that test.

Also note that in the U.S. our average daily calorie consumption has gone up by 150 calories (women) to 300 calories (men) over the last few decades. I've seen published estimates even higher: 400–500 calories. If that doesn't seem like much to you, trust me that when accumulated over the years, it's surprising that we're not fatter than we are.

15

HOW COMMON IS DIABETES?

In the U.S. as of 2014, 29 million Americans had diabetes, including 11% of all adults. Eight of the 29 million didn't even know they had it. The risk of type 2 diabetes rises with age, to the point that one in four over 65 has diabetes. Based on hemoglobin A1c levels, another 86 million adults in the U.S. have prediabetes: that's one out of every three adults. Of those over age 65, half have prediabetes and less than one in 10 know they have it. These figures are from the U.S. Centers for Disease Control.

It's difficult to measure, but the U.S. probably has about three million type 1 diabetics. Two hundred thousand of those are under age 20.

Of course, the diabetes epidemic is not just a U.S. problem. The prevalence of diabetes across the globe has doubled in the last three decades. Almost one in 10 adults worldwide has diabetes, mostly type 2. Here are the current prevalence rates of adult diabetes in selected countries: United Kingdom 6%, New Zealand 9%, Canada 9%, India 9%, Australia 10%, United States 11%, and Mexico 16%. Many Middle East countries exceed 15%.

We're even starting to see type 2 diabetes in children, which was quite rare just thirty years ago. It's undoubtedly related to overweight and obesity. Childhood obesity has more than doubled in U.S. children and quadrupled in adolescents in the last 30 years. Looking at children aged 6–11 years, 18% are obese. The obesity rate for adolescents aged 12–19 years is 21%. Obesity and overweight together describe 32% of U.S. children.

The prevalence of diabetes and prediabetes in U.S. adolescents increased from 9% in 1999 to 23% in 2008.

MEDICAL COMPLICATIONS OF DIABETES

Diabetes is important because it has the potential to damage many different organ systems, degrading quality of life. It can damage nerves (neuropathy), eyes (retinopathy), kidneys (nephropathy), and stomach function (gastroparesis). Diabetics are at higher risk for periodontal (gum) disease, depression, and lower limb amputations.

Just as important, diabetes can cut life short. It's the seventh leading cause of death in the U.S. Compared to those who are free of diabetes, having diabetes at age 50 more than doubles the risk of developing cardiovascular disease: heart attacks, strokes, and high blood pressure. Compared to those without diabetes, having both cardiovascular disease and diabetes approximately doubles the risk of dying. Compared to those without diabetes, women and men with diabetes at age 50 die seven or eight years earlier, on average.

Diabetic complications and survival rates will undoubtedly improve over the coming years as we learn how to better treat this disease.

TESTIMONIALS

(Source references used in this book will be numbered sequentially in parentheses and listed in the "References" section of the Appendix.)

17

Dave Wendel, a type 1 diabetic, shared his experience with the Paleolithic diet at Robb Wolf's website in 2011 (1). Dave used Wolf's "Paleo Solution." At first, Dave was terrified by the thought of giving up his beloved carbohydrates, pizza, beer, and bread, for example. On the other hand, he thought carbohydrates were probably why Americans kept getting fatter. His blood sugars were like a roller coaster. Once he reduced his carb intake, he discovered he didn't miss them. By replacing carbs with proteins and good fats, he didn't suffer the hunger that can lead to binge eating. Before starting the program, his daily carb intake was 100–200 grams and his average insulin dose was 37–48 units, with 24 of those as basal dosing (long-acting insulin). After starting the new diet, he cut his carbs to "almost nothing," and his blood glucose levels dropped from 250–300 mg/dl or higher (14–17mmol/l) to 80–120 mg/dl (4.4–6.7 mmol/l). He was able to reduce his insulin by almost half, to 24 units a day. This occurred over three weeks. He started feeling better than he had in years.

Ray Audette reported a cure of both his rheumatoid arthritis and diabetes (presumably type 2) via the Paleolithic diet (2). *Dallas Observer News* had an article on him in 1995. A quote: "It's a lifestyle through which Audette swears he has shed 25 pounds [11 kg], transformed a flabby body into a tight mass of sinew, and, perhaps most impressively, cured his own serious medical maladies— rheumatoid arthritis and diabetes. Audette's guiding principle is simple: Do what the cavemen did. If Stone Age man couldn't have speared whatever culinary delight you're about to pop into your mouth or if the Neanderthal couldn't have plucked it off a bush, Audette argues you should avoid it, too." Read more about Mr. Audette's experience in his book *Neanderthin.*

A blogger named Rich wrote of his success with the paleo diet in 2012 at his "Rich the Diabetic" blog (3). Rich is a type 1 who was diagnosed at the age of a year-and-a-half. The paleo lifestyle led to a 2.5 point drop in his hemoglobin A1c in just six months. For those unfamiliar, hemoglobin A1c is a measure of blood sugar control; a drop of 2.5 points means his blood sugars were about 100 mg/dl (5.6 mmol/l) lower after starting the diet. Before starting his paleo journey, Rich's hemoglobin A1c was an embarrassing 11.4. Before going paleo, he "used to live on cereals, tv dinners, potato chips, cookies, microwavable meals, fast food, pizza, etc." He plans on staying paleo for life. Here's how he summarizes his lifestyle: "It's pretty simple, eat like our hunter gatherer ancestors, exercise like them, get outdoors, and reduce your carbs. Most people these days eat anywhere between 200–300 carbs [grams] a day, and some eat even more! On paleo I've been averaging around 100 carbs a day....I buy whole foods (fruits and lots of veggies), a little frozen veggies for convenience and storage time, lots of meat, no dairy, and lots of olive and coconut oil. I cook a lot now, which means I do a lot more dishes than I want to, but it's been worth it."

Dr. Stephan Guyenet in 2012 interviewed C. Vicky Beer, M.D., about her experience with the paleo diet in her patients, diabetic or not (4). Dr. Beer commented about people with diabetes specifically:

"Every patient I have ever had with diabetes who has adhered to the paleo diet for most of the time has experienced dramatic results. Every one of them has been able to reduce their blood sugars and reduce their medications significantly, and in some instances, stop their medicine altogether. This is not unlike other more known popular diets such as

South Beach or Zone, which are actually quite similar to the Paleo diet in composition."

Steve Cooksey is a middle-aged type 2 diabetic who had a blood glucose in excess of 700 mg/dl (39 mmol/l) at the time of his diagnosis, when he spent four days in the hospital (5). After initially improving on a low-glycemic-index diet, Steve moved to a low-carb paleo diet inspired by Mark Sisson's Primal Blueprint. He also abandoned his sedentary ways. Relatively quickly, he dropped his weight from 235 to 165 pounds (107 to 75 kg), was able to stop his insulin and Actos (pioglitazone), moved his cholesterol from high to normal, and his weekly acid reflux and indigestion flare-ups went into remission.

Dr. Ernie Garcia in Louisiana wrote this at his blog (PaleolithicMD.com) in 2012 (6). "I became quite frustrated as traditional "diabetic" diets seemed useless at improving LONGTERM control of a patient's disease process....I have had many diabetics commit to a Paleo lifestyle, and the results have been remarkable....I see Paleo as an alternative for patients to keep their blood sugars lower with LESS medicine! In the end, only one thing matters...get those sugars down. Paleo adds another weapon in the arsenal....Again, with my diabetics I sit down and explain why I feel Paleo will benefit them. I do this in detail, and utilize some simple handouts I've written up as to how making the right food choices can truly help control blood sugar. I then discuss the experiences my other patients have had after adapting their lifestyle. I make it perfectly clear that in my opinion, their best chance for long term sugar control and limiting the meds they will need to use is to adapt an 85-90% Paleolithic lifestyle....There are many applications of the Paleo diet to chronic disease, but my passion at the moment has to do with it's application in the diabetic population.

From the hormonal standpoint it strikes at the core of the disease, and offers AMAZING potential for REAL change in people's lives."

Amanda Torres shares her story at her blog, The Curious Coconut (7). She followed Mark Sisson's Primal Blueprint version of the paleo diet. In 2009, Amanda was 25 years old and weighed 210 lb (95 kg). At 65 inches tall (165 cm), that gave her a body mass index of 34.9, solidly in the obese range. She was taking two antidepressants, anti-anxiety pills, sleeping pills, periodic Prilosec (a stomach acid reducer), frequent antacids, and occasional antidiarrhea pills. She was prone to respiratory infections and frequently needed antibiotics. She suffered from rosacea, acne, and worst of all, hidradenitis suppurativa [pustules and carbuncles mostly in the armpits]. She had frequent yeast and urinary tract infections. As if that weren't enough, in 2008 she had been diagnosed with prediabetes, metabolic syndrome and high blood pressure. She figures she was a full-blown type 2 diabetic by the end of 2009. She was justifiably scared about her long-term prospects. After doing her due diligence, Amanda took the plunge into her new lifestyle at the start of 2010. She lost 80 lb (36 kg) in the first year. Three years out, she still weighs 140 lb (64 kg). Additionally, she noted major improvements in her gastrointestinal ailments, improved mood and mental clarity, better sleep, much less acne, and immediate relief of hidradenitis suppurativa. Amanda's blood pressure returned to normal as did her insulin sensitivity.

Dietitian Kelly Schmidt has a blog, Paleo Infused Nutrition, at which she has published several interviews with diabetics eating a Paleolithic diet. First up is an interview with an adult-onset type 1 diabetic, Alexis, who follows a low-carb "primal" eating pattern (8). Alexis noted improved overall health, better mood, healthier hair and fingernails, and much clearer skin. Her dental health is dramatically improved, with fewer cavities and less need for professional cleaning

Kelly Schmidt also published a blog interview with Intrepid Pioneer, who has LADA—Latent Autoimmune Diabetes of Adulthood (9). LADA is much closer to type 1 than type 2 diabetes, so he's on insulin. Intrepid Pioneer's paleo diet was inspired initially by a "Whole 30 Challenge." He makes room for cheese and home-brewed beer; so he's not pure paleo. Intrepid Pioneer was diagnosed with diabetes in May, 2011, during a routine annual physical. His blood sugars ran around 360 mg/dl (20 mmol/l), with a hemoglobin A1c of 12.3. Since adopting the paleo lifestyle, he's been able to mostly stop his rapid-acting mealtime insulin; he uses it only for treats like pizza or Thanksgiving dinner. He was able to reduce his long-acting insulin dose by over 10 units. Intrepid told Kelly that, "Paleo is great and it all tastes so good because it's real food, but I have found that I also need to exercise, eating Paleo combined with exercise has yielded dynamic results. My endocrinologist was blown away by all that I had done, reduced my insulin injections and basically had my A1C's in check—my last appointment I was 7.3. Still a bit more to go but the last time I was pushing 9 just six months before."

Kelly Schmidt strikes yet again with an interview with Shelby Hughes, who was diagnosed at age 39 with type 1 diabetes (10). Before going paleo, Shelby had tried a low-carb diet, which did improve her blood sugars. However, she couldn't sustain the diet over the long run. She fell off the wagon, returned to the Standard American Diet (SAD), and boarded the blood sugar rollercoaster. At the start of 2013,

Shelby started the paleo lifestyle for a two-week trial. She reports that, "After two weeks, I noticed that my blood sugars were AMAZINGLY stable. I didn't have lows, I didn't have highs. I never looked back!....My sleep has improved....I have lost weight, but I think that's mainly because I'm staying within or just below my caloric requirements and I've increased my exercise. But I do have tons of energy."

Gary Rea was 55 when he was diagnosed with type 2 diabetes: blood glucose 218 mg/dl (12 mmol/l) (11). He started on Loren Cordain's version of the paleo diet and over the course of a year lost weight from 235 to 160 pounds (107 to 73 kg), dropped his high blood pressure from 180/90 to 115/72, and cut his triglycerides from high down to the normal range. He believes his diabetes is cured. (I'd be a bit more cautious and say "in remission.")

Lindsay Swanson shared her experience with the Paleolithic diet at the Joslin Diabetes Blog (12). She was diagnosed with type 1 diabetes at age 25. Lindsay's initial interest was spurred by years of undiagnosed gastrointestinal issues. She eased into the Paleolithic diet by sequentially eliminating certain food classes, starting with grains, then soy, then other legumes. As she did, she felt increasingly better. Lindsay eats few refined carbohydrates. My sense is she doesn't require much insulin. She wrote, "Much to my surprise, my blood sugars completely leveled out, so much so that I rarely need to treat a low blood sugar, and spikes are few and far between....Probably 75 percent of my diet consists of vegetables and plant based food, some with more carbohydrates depending on my activity level. I eat a lot of fat/protein regularly, examples: avocados, coconut oil (in tea and cooking), grassfed meats, bacon (and the reserved fat), oils, nuts, etc."

Dr. Keith R. Runyan (M.D.) is an internist, nephrologist, and obesity medicine specialist (13). He was diagnosed with type 1 diabetes at the age of 36. He has combined a low-carb ketogenic diet with the Paleolithic diet to fuel his athletic lifestyle and better control his diabetes. At his website, he writes that "...the treatment of diabetes should begin with restricting carbohydrate, the most insulin requiring macronutrient that is at the same time, nonessential to human existence." Dr. Runyan notes that many type 2 diabetics have both limited insulin-secreting capacity and resistance to insulin action. In such a setting, he sees that restricting dietary carbohydrates improves blood glucose levels and, over time, improves insulin sensitivity. He personally had very disappointing results with the standard diabetic diet. Since adopting his new diet in 2012, he's noticed much better blood sugar control, fewer episodes of low blood sugar, and he needs less insulin (just 20 units a day when exercising regularly). So what does Dr. Runyan eat?

- "The protein in my diet comes from grass-fed beef, lamb, and pork (which is higher in omega-3 fatty acids than grain-fed), fish (primarily wild caught Alaska salmon), nuts & seeds (primarily macadamia, pistachio, and pumpkin seeds)."
- "Fat in my diet primarily comes from meat, beef tallow, lamb lard, eggs, fish, nuts, coconut oil, olives and olive oil."
- "Carbohydrates in my diet come from non-starchy vegetables (kale, collard greens, yellow squash, zucchini squash, brussels sprouts, lettuce, etc), and the small amount of carbohydrates contained in nuts, and 2 tbsp [30 ml] lemon juice for salads. I avoid all grains and foods made from grains, fruits (except tomato and avocado), potatoes, and legumes."

Dr. Runyan designed his very-low-carb Paleolithic diet based on the ideas of Loren Cordain, Ph.D. (except he includes more fat and avoids fruit except for occasional berries) and Richard K. Bernstein, M,D., Stephen Phinney, M.D., Ph.D., Jeff Volek, R.D., Ph.D., and Eric Westman, M.D., which he believes is optimal for those with diabetes. He aims to limit carbohydrate consumption to 50 grams a day or less.

Robert Oh, M.D., a family physician with the U.S. Army, was diagnosed with prediabetes when in his late 30s (14). He has no family history of diabetes. Prior to his diagnosis, he was quite physically active with a type of high-intensity training called Cross-Fit. Paleolithic-style eating, by the way, is very popular among CrossFitters. Furthermore, Dr. Oh's body mass index was solidly in the healthy range at 23. He did have one apparent risk factor for diabetes: he was taking a statin drug to lower his cholesterol level. After stopping the statin and instituting Robb Wolf's version of the paleo diet, he quickly saw a return of his blood sugar levels (via a hemoglobin A1c test) to normal. Dr. Oh believes the diet change was key to his improvement.

IT'S NOT FOR EVERYONE

Allison Nimlos is a type 1 PWD (person with diabetes). She tried the "Whole 30" version of the Paleolithic Diet in 2013 and shared her experience at her blog, The Blood Sugar Whisperer (15). After a three-month trial, she found the Paleolithic diet unsustainable. It was too restrictive; she felt deprived. Dining out was her biggest downfall; she ordered whatever she wanted, admitting that it had adverse effects on her blood sugar. She also buys a lot of ice cream, which is not a caveman food. Allison did notice her blood sugars and hemoglobin A1c improved "quite a bit" during her trial. She noticed that she tended to eat less, attributing that to the satiating effect of relatively high protein consumption. The diet did lower her carbohydrate intake, resulting in less blood sugar fluctuations. In her experience, "there is a direct relationship between more carbohydrates and a more difficult to manage diabetes...." Although she doesn't consider herself a paleo dieter these days, she and her husband still cook many paleo meals at home because they're delicious. I have nothing against the "Whole 30" program; it's a good paleo-style eating plan that is healthier than the standard American and most diabetic diets. I'm sure there are diabetics who have improved their health and blood sugar levels with the Whole 30 plan.

I am indebted to these patients and physicians for sharing their Paleolithic diet experiences with the world. Could these testimonials reflect unintentional "cherry-picking," i.e., reporting primarily good experiences and sweeping the bad under the carpet? I suppose so. As of this writing, I honestly can't recall off-hand hearing about a patient having a poor physical outcome and therefore abandoning the Paleolithic diet. But it's probably happened. Paleo diet "failures" are more likely to be similar to those eating very-low-carb to control diabetes: the siren songs of refined sugars and grains and over-processed foods are hard to resist in our carb-centric culture.

HOUSEKEEPING

While reading the testimonials above, you likely noticed that the Paleolithic diet isn't monolithic: several versions exist (16). It was the same in antiquity.

We don't have many scientific clinical studies looking at the Paleolithic diet in diabetics. The few that we have are discussed in the Appendix; see "Scientific Support for a Paleo-Style Diabetic Diet". You may also enjoy an Appendix section called "Newer Theories on the Cause of Type 2 Diabetes." I put both of those sections in the Appendix because they won't be of much interest to readers without a biomedical or scientific background.

Also in the Appendix, don't miss the list of helpful "Additional Resources" and "Definitions of Diabetes, Prediabetes, and Gestational Diabetes."

As mentioned previously, source references used in this book are numbered sequentially in parentheses and listed in the "References" section of the Appendix.

About a decade ago, some in the diabetes community started using the term PWD, "person with diabetes." Or people with diabetes. The idea is that calling someone "a diabetic" reduces him to a stereotype, oversimplifying the situation and diminishing the person with diabetes. The same would be true for labeling someone asthmatic, alcoholic, or epileptic. In my experience, a majority of persons with diabetes still haven't heard of PWD, so for clarity's sake I will use "diabetic" in this book. I love acronyms, so I'll switch over to PWD when most folks know what it means. Trust me, physicians and nurses use "diabetics" all the time, not "PWDs." We mean no disrespect by it.

Throughout this book, the use of "I" or "my" or "me," will typically refer to Steve Parker, M.D., the principal author. "We" or "our" refers to both Steve and his co-author wife, Sunny Parker. Sunny served primarily as the editor, food maven, recipe mastermind, and Steve's muse. "The Parker Compound" is our secret underground bunker in Arizona, USA.

If you faithfully adhere to the Paleobetic Diet for several weeks or months, I'd love to get feedback from you. Did it lower your blood sugars? Did you lose any excess weight? Did you have hypoglycemic episodes or other adverse effects? Did you see changes in your blood pressure or lipids (cholesterols and triglycerides)? Were you able to reduce your diabetic drugs? If you aim to lose weight, consider taking before and after photos. You can reach me via e-mail at steveparkermd@gmail.com. I won't share your personal information with anyone unless I have your consent. Also feel free also to share your experience at various online diabetes forums.

I would be much obliged if you left a review of the book at Amazon.com and similar venues. I'm convinced that the Paleobetic Diet is a healthful way of eating. Would you help me spread the word?

2
Early Human History

THE INTERSECTION OF EVOLUTIONARY THEORY AND RELIGION

If you don't believe in evolution or don't have any interest in the history of early man (paleoanthropology), you can skip this first section. Much of what follows is controversial and isn't subject to scientific investigation.

Most religions address the origin of *Homo sapiens* (that's us) in some way. For instance, some fundamentalist Christians believe that God created the universe, Earth, and life over the course of six days about six thousand years ago. Many other Christians disagree.

The scientific fields of geology, archeology, and paleontology suggest that the Earth and its life are indeed older than 6,000 years. Much older. Four and a half billion years older. Fossilized remains of organisms indicate that some animal and plant species living millions of years ago are no longer with us. Dinosaurs, for example, mostly died out 66 million years ago. (Birds may be their direct descendants.)

I have a college degree in Zoology, so I was thoroughly indoctrinated in Charles Darwin's evolutionary theory, at least the version current in the mid-1970s. Very few biologists doubt that evolution occurred and still occurs. Darwin's theory requires no God, or didn't include a role for God or gods. It doesn't address the question of Creation.

Scientists tell us the Paleolithic Era started 2.5 million years ago and ended about 10,000 years ago. It includes the evolution of hominins (our pre-human ancestors) at the start of the Paleolithic and, later, humans (starting about 200,000 years ago). The Paleolithic is also called Old Stone Age because it's characterized by the use of stone tools by early man and our hominin ancestors. Let's assume there hasn't been much additional human genetic change (evolution) over the last 50,000 years.

The cornerstone of paleo-style eating is that we should eat the things we are evolutionarily adapted to eat. We'll be healthier that way. We didn't have corn chips, soda pop, and candy bars 20,000 years ago, so we shouldn't be eating them now. Our bodies aren't designed to handle them, certainly not in the quantities we consume now. It's an evolutionary mismatch.

Sounds reasonable, doesn't it? Various species of animals thrive on certain foods and not others. My horses eat two meals a day—all hay. You and I couldn't survive on that. (Ideally, the horses would graze all day long, but the Parker Compound doesn't have pastures.) Our bodies thrive on certain foods and not others. That's true for all animals. The range of foods humans can survive on is pretty broad. Whether the optimal way of eating is determined by godless evolutionary processes or by the intelligent design of a Creator doesn't matter if you're looking at it from a purely nutritional viewpoint.

From an "everlasting life" viewpoint, it matters.

Christianity and the Paleolithic diet theory are not mutually exclusive. A Christian can simply ignore the possibility of millions of years of evolution, believing instead that God made our bodies in such a way that we'd be healthier eating certain foods and not others. Those foods may be the components of the Paleolithic diet, whatever that is.

(I don't know where Judaism, Hinduism, Islam, Buddhism, Shinto, and other major religions stand on evolution. You google it.)

Many proponents of evolutionary theory are atheist or agnostic. In their view, "natural selection" determines who lives or dies, not the hand of God. If you haven't evolved the necessary adaptations to survive and reproduce in a particular environment, you die. In his autobiography, Charles Darwin wrote, "Another source of conviction in the existence of God, connected with the reason and not with the feelings, impresses me as having much more weight. This follows from the extreme difficulty or rather impossibility of conceiving this immense and wonderful universe, including man with his capacity of looking far backwards and far into futurity, as the result of blind chance or necessity. When thus reflecting I feel compelled to look to a First Cause having an

31

intelligent mind in some degree analogous to that of man; and I deserve to be called a Theist."

In case you're wondering, I'm a Christian. This simply means I believe I was given life by God, that His son Jesus became a man and died for my sins, and that I will have everlasting life in heaven for believing this (17). I strive to live the way God would want me to live, as written in the Holy Bible. I readily admit that I often fail to meet God's expectations—that's what sin is—but I vow to do better. I was brought up in the Catholic faith, even attending parochial school in grades 1–8, but I'm Protestant now. I went through an agnostic period from the age 19 to about 38; by God's grace I made it through that alive.

I believe God created us, all life, and the universe. There's no proof; it's a matter of faith. I don't know if He made humans 6,000 years ago or 200,000. The bulk of the scientific evidence is clearly against 6,000 years ago. Perhaps God actually made the Earth and universe 6,000 years ago, putting in place misleading geological and paleontological evidence at the same time as a Divine joke.

I wonder if God made Adam and Eve 200,000 years ago, and *Homo habilis*, *Homo erectus*, and our other hominin "ancestors" are just extinct animals like the dodo bird and dinosaurs.

HUMAN EVOLUTION AND MIGRATION

Evolutionary theory holds that we humans (*Homo sapiens*) evolved from non-human primates (hominins) in a process that started about 2.5 million years ago in Africa. Prominent ancestors include *Homo habilis* (2.3 million years ago) and *Homo erec-*

tus (1.8 million years ago). *Homo sapiens* eventually hit the scene 200,000 years ago, probably in east Africa, which is considered the cradle of humanity. (All Americans can honestly fill out forms that ask for our race as "African-American.") The paleoanthropologists tell us we share many genetic traits with long-extinct hominins from two million years ago.

We have evidence of behaviorally modern humans from about 50,000 years ago, if not longer. In other words, in addition to looking like us, they acted like us.

The "Out of Africa" hypothesis to explain the worldwide spread of humans says that *Homo sapiens* arose in Africa, then began migrating between 50,000 and 100,000 years ago. A competing "multiregional" hypothesis involves *Homo erectus* dispersing to many regions throughout Africa, Europe, and Asia, then somehow interbreeding and culminating in *Homo sapiens* in several regions. *Homo erectus* may have begun to spread out of Africa as long as 1.4 million years ago. Among the experts, the Out of Africa theory is currently favored over the multiregional hypothesis.

Starting roughly 100,000 years ago, anatomically modern humans began migrating out of Africa, into the Near East. By 50,000 years ago we were into South Asia, then Australia 40 or 50,000 years ago. We spread to Europe 40,000 years ago. Northeast Asians moved into North America (Alaska) 12 to 30,000 years ago; South America followed.

At this point, we've made it to every spot on Earth that can support life. We've even gone to the moon.

As points of reference, the Bronze Age started 5,500 years ago in the Near East and the earliest known writing was 5,000 years ago.

EXTRA CREDIT FOR SCIENCE NERDS: THE PACE OF HUMAN EVOLUTION

Most paleo lifestyle proponents think that, genetically speaking, those of us living today are pretty much the same as our ancestors living 50,000 or even 200,000 thousand years ago. That may not be the case.

This traditional view of the rate of human evolution's is articulated by Artemis P. Simopoulos, who was with The Center for Genetics, Nutrition and Health in 2009 when he wrote:

"The spontaneous mutation rate for nuclear DNA is estimated at 0.5% per million years. Therefore, over the past 10,000 years there has been time for very little change in our genes, perhaps 0.005%. In fact, our genes today are very similar to the genes of our ancestors during the Paleolithic period 40,000 years ago, at which time our genetic profile was established."

On the other hand, the experts are debating now whether the pace of human evolution has accelerated over the last 10,000 years. The iconoclasts say it has. For example, note that most mammals lose the ability to digest milk after they've been weaned off the teat in early life: they lose the lactase enzyme that allowed them to digest milk sugar (lactose). That's why lactose intolerance is so common among adult humans—only a third of us worldwide can digest milk. Between 5,000 and 10,000 years ago, a genetic mutation occurred that allowed those possessing the new gene to consume and digest milk.

So a whole new source of food for adults opened up: dairy cattle. Would that have conferred a survival advantage? You bet. We have evidence that the milk-digesting mutation spread fairly quickly since its appearance. But it hasn't spread across the globe uniformly. The ability to digest milk in adulthood—called lactase persistence—is less than 40% in Greece and Turkey, but higher than 90% in the UK and Scandinavia.

Another oft-cited example of rapid and recent human evolution is the appearance and spread of blue eyes starting 6,000 to 10,000 years ago. Everyone with blue eyes today apparently has a common ancestor that had a gene mutation back then, when everybody had brown eyes.

For more information on the "rapid evolution" idea, check out the writings of Gregory Cochran, Henry Harpending, and John Hawks. Also consider a new book by Nicholas Wade, "A Troublesome Inheritance: Genes, Race, and Human History." Wade is a science writer for the *New York Times*.

DIET IMPLICATIONS OF HUMAN ORIGINS AND MIGRATION

Until 10,000 or 12,000 or so years ago, humans and our hominin ancestors obtained food through a combination of hunting and foraging. We hunted small or large game and birds. At some point we learned how to catch fish and shellfish. We searched for and gathered up fruits, berries, leafy plants, nuts, seeds, mussels, clams, honey, eggs, and roots. The range of edible items expanded when we harnessed the power of fire for cooking, which was at least 230,000 years ago and may have been as long as a million years ago. Tools and weapons also expanded our possibilities from the very start of the Paleolithic. At this point, prior to 10,000 years ago, we weren't farming or raising cattle and dairy cows.

Available foods depended on local climatic conditions, soil, and water availability. Climate, in turn, is heavily dependent on latitude (how far away from the equator) and altitude. East Africa at the dawn of humanity is described as savanna: grass-filled plains with scattered patches of forest, and relatively dry. Plants and animals available there would be much different than the colder but wetter Europe 200,000 years ago. Humans in Northern Europe tended to eat more animal-based food and relatively less plant matter than savanna-dwellers, perhaps just because there were fewer edible plants growing in the cold climate.

Many plants would have been highly seasonal, just as they are now. Tribes of humans walked or migrated to nearby micro-climates as one plant went out of season and another came into season. Tribes followed prey animals as they also migrated in search of seasonal food.

Due to technological limitations, we wouldn't have been able to utilize some potential food sources that required much processing, such as cereal grains and legumes. Since we weren't yet pastoralists (raising sheep, cattle, etc.), we would have access to milk only if we killed a nursing prey animal. Have you ever tried to milk a wild water buffalo? Not advisable. Ability to digest milk was marginal. Even today, two-thirds of humans lose the ability to digest milk after infancy.

The experts are debating how long we've been consuming significant amounts of cereal grains and roots. Canadian researchers working in Africa suggest we've enjoyed them for over 100,000 years (18).

WHAT DOES THE PALEOLITHIC DIET LOOK LIKE?

It's quite difficult to know exactly what early humans ate 100,000 years ago. Scientists use a variety of methods to investigate, including analysis of patterns of wear on teeth, searches of prehistoric dwellings, and analysis of carbon isotopes in organic matter. Some of the best-preserved human prehistoric artifacts are found in caves, which protected them from environmental degradation. That's why the paleo diet is sometimes called the caveman diet. We have an inkling of what foods were available in specific climates and regions. We have some ideas about tools our ancestors had available to hunt, gather, and process foods. Perhaps most reliably, we have fairly good data on what modern hunter-gatherer groups eat (for those few still in existence) or ate (for those lately extinct or modernized).

SUMMARY: THE PALEOLITHIC VERSUS TYPICAL MODERN WESTERN DIET

Today we get most of our calories from grains, sugars, domesticated livestock, and dairy products. On the other hand, our pre-agricultural ancestors ate primarily wild game and naturally occurring plant foods. Their carbohydrates would have come from fruits and vegetables rather than cereal grains, diary products, and refined sugars. They ate no junk food, no industrial seed oils, and very few grains and dairy products. Compared to us, they ate more potassium, fiber, protein, and micronutrients, but less sodium and carbohydrate. They ate relatively more omega-3 fatty acids and less omega-6s.

Paleo dieters today aim to consume natural whole foods while minimizing simple sugars and refined starches. The paleo community generally is convinced that grains and legumes are harmful, while others disagree. Dairy products are allowed in some versions of paleo, although purists would vote against.

Now let's dig into the details.

THE EATON AND KONNER MODEL

S. Boyd Eaton and Melvin Konner in 2010 looked carefully at the diet of pre-industrial hunter-gatherers and proposed a prototypical ancestral diet (20). Again, remember that actual diet would vary with climate, latitude, altitude, water availability, etc. Eaton and Konner suggest our ancestral diet looked like this:

- Carbohydrates: 35–40% of daily energy (calories)
- Protein: 25–30% of daily energy
- Fat: 20–35% of daily energy
- Added sugar: 2% of daily energy
- Fiber: over 70 g/day
- EPA and DHA*: 0.7–6 g/day
- Cholesterol: 500+ mg/day
- Vitamin C: 500 mg/day
- Vitamin D: 4,000 IU/day (from sunlight)
- Calcium: 1,000–1,500 mg/day
- Sodium: under 1,000 mg/day
- Potassium: 7,000 mg/day

*Eicosapentaenoic acid and docosahexaenoic acid (omega-3 fatty acids)

Their conception of a modern Paleolithic food pyramid is a base of high-fiber vegetables and fruits, the next tier up being meat/fish/low-fat dairy (all lean), then a possible tier for whole grain (admittedly very unusual), with a small peak of oils, fats, and refined carbohydrates. Their inclusion of dairy products and whole grains must be a concession to convenience and the reality that those items can be healthful for modern humans.

Eaton and Konner note that hunter-gatherer groups had a high degree of dependence on plant foods, while obtaining 35 to 65% of diet (calories rather than weight, I assume) from animal flesh. They found some modern hunter-gatherer cultures deriving as much as 65% of calories from carbohydrate (mostly plants, then). It's a mistake to assume that the typical Paleolithic diet is necessarily meat-based, as the popular press so often describes it.

Eaton and Konner make a few other distinctions that are worth mentioning now. Game animals have more mono- and polyunsaturated fatty acids than supermarket meat. The Paleolithic diet's ratio of omega-6 to omega-3 fatty acids was about 2:1, in contrast to the modern Western ratio of 10:1 or even higher.

I'd like to share a few more tidbits from their 2010 article:
- The transition from hunting/gathering to farming (about 10,000 year ago) saw a decrease in body size and robustness, plus evidence of nutritional stress.
- Levels of muscular and aerobic fitness in ancestral groups are much higher than modern societies, with a concomitant higher level of calorie consumption.

- Average life expectancies in pre-industrial hunter-gatherer (H-G) groups was only 30–35 years, but much of this low number simply reflects high infant and child death rates.
- H-G deaths overwhelmingly reflect infectious diseases.
- H-G groups had a high degree of dependence on plant foods.
- Fish and shellfish are more important food sources than these authors had estimated 25 years earlier.
- H-G diets are higher in fat and protein than they once thought.
- Nearly all H-G carbs are from vegetables and fruits, which have more favorable glycemic responses (i.e., a lesser rise in blood sugar) than grains and concentrated sugars.
- Uncultivated or wild fruits and vegetables have much more fiber than commercial ones (13 versus 4 g fiber per 100 g of food).

The Diet-Heart Hypothesis is the idea that dietary total and saturated fat, and cholesterol, cause or contribute to atherosclerosis (hardening of the arteries), leading to heart attacks and strokes. Konner and Eaton still believe (in 2010 at least) the theory is valid for fats, but not cholesterol. The latest evidence, however, is that total and saturated fat are minimally, if at all, related to atherosclerosis (19).

They also believe total fat, due to its caloric load, is an important contributor to obesity and type 2 diabetes. I agree that may be true, especially if you eat a lot of carbohydrates with fat.

To further imitate the Paleolithic lifestyle, Eaton and Konner also recommend high activity levels, including resistance exercise, flexibility, aerobics, and burning over 1,000 calories daily exclusive of resting metabolism.

But let's not put all our eggs in the Eaton and Konner basket.

THE KUIPERS MODEL

A 2010 scientific article by Kuipers et al suggests that the East African Paleolithic diet derived, on average, 25–29% of calories from protein, 30–39% from fat, and 39–40% from carbohydrate (21). That qualifies as mildly low-carb, and similar to Eaton and Konner's macronutrient breakdown. Modern Western percentages for protein, fat, and carb are 15%, 33%, and 50%, respectively. Kuipers et al suggest that the evolution of our large brains in East Africa may have been possible by utilization of aquatic resources such as fish, lobster, crab, shrimp, sea urchins, squid, octopus, and amphibians. Rather than savannah, this was a land-water ecosytem. Diets here would have been rich in the omega-3 fatty acids we find in fish oil (EPA and DHA). Kuipers believes roots and tubers were also part of the Paleolithic diet.

THE CORDAIN MODEL

Loren Cordain and associates in 2000 suggested that Paleolithic diets derived about a third—22 to 40%—of calories from carbohydrate, based on modern hunter-gatherer societies (22). The lower carb consumption compared to Western diets left more room for moderate to high amounts of protein and fat. Dr. Cordain is a co-author with Eaton and Konner on many paleo diet scientific articles, so they don't have many differences.

Dr. Cordain (Ph.D.) is probably the preeminent scientist who advocates the Paleolithic diet. He's made a few modifications in his model diet over the years. From his website in 2014, the following are the seven pillars of his conception of the modern paleo diet compared to the typical Western diet (23). The paleo diet is:

- higher in protein (25–30% of calories versus 15%)
- lower in carbohydrates and glycemic index via nonstarchy fresh fruits and vegetables
- higher in fiber
- moderate to high fat content, especially monounsaturated fats and polyunsaturated fats (particularly omega-3 fatty acids)
- higher in potassium and lower in sodium
- higher dietary alkaline load relative to acid load (vegetables and fruit counteract the acid in meat and fish)
- higher in many vitamins, minerals, antioxidants and plant phytochemicals

CARBOHYDRATE CONTENT OF THE PALEO DIET

Since dietary carbohydrates are major contributors to blood sugar, the carbohydrates in the Paleolithic diet are important. It appears that the average paleo diet derived about a third of calories from carbohydrate: that qualifies as low-carb since the average Western diet provides half of calories as carbohydrate. The carbohydrates eaten by Paleolithic man were accompanied by lots of fiber, over four times as much as the average American diet (70+ grams versus 15 grams). The sources of carbohydrate were fruits, vegetables, and roots or tubers, with minimal and seasonal contribution from honey. Fiber is important since high consumption is linked in modern times to lower rates of type 2 diabetes, and fiber also slows and limits the rise in blood sugar after meals. Furthermore, the original Paleolithic carbohydrate sources generally would have been much less calorically dense than modern carbohydrates sources. For instance, one Frosted Strawberry Pop-Tart has the same amount of calories (200) as four cups of fresh strawberry halves, but the Pop-Tart has less than one gram of fiber compared to 12 gm in the raw berries.

Because of our modification of edible plants and animals through selective breeding and genetic modification, it's impossible for most of us to accurately recreate the diet of our Paleolithic ancestors. The closest you could come would be to live entirely off the land, catching or hunting wild animals and foraging for wild plants. That's a heck of a lot of work, and wouldn't sustain more than a tiny fraction of the planet's current seven billion souls.

If we're going to construct a modern Paleolithic-style diet, now we've got some anchoring numbers.

If this book must be dedicated to someone, it should be to the occasional man, woman, or child who still can resist the specious authority of food merchants, their lavish advertisements and spectacular television commercials, and retain sufficient intellectual independence to think for themselves.

—Walter L. Voegtlin, M.D., in *The Stone Age Diet* (1975)

3
Out of Eden: The Neolithic Period and Beyond

With the advent of the Agricultural Revolution 10,000 years ago, mankind took a giant leap away from two million years of evolutionary adaptation. The Industrial Revolution that started in the late 18th century—about 240 years ago—was yet another watershed event.

The Agricultural Revolution marks the end of the Old Stone Age and the start of the Neolithic period. The Neolithic ended four to six thousand years ago, replaced by the Bronze Age (or Iron Age in some areas).

EFFECTS OF THE AGRICULTURAL REVOLUTION

The Agricultural Revolution refers to farming the land on a large scale, and all that entails: gathering and planting seeds, nurturing the soil, breeding plants for desirable traits, storing crops, processing plants to maximize digestibility, domesticating wild animals and enhancing them by selective breeding, setting down roots in one geographic location, etc.

The revolution allowed for the expansion of reliable food supplies and an explosion of human populations. Less time was needed for hunting and foraging, allowing for the development of advanced cultures.

It wasn't all sunshine and roses, however. We have evidence that human health deteriorated as a result of the revolution. For instance, some populations declined in height and dental health.

EFFECTS OF THE INDUSTRIAL REVOLUTION

The Industrial Revolution starting in the late 18th century brought its own changes to our diet. Progressive industrialization and affluence changed the composition of our "energy foods." For instance, peasants in poor developing countries derive about 75% of their calories from high-fiber starchy foods. With modernization, fiber-free fats and sugars become the source of 60% of calories. U.S. consumption of cereal fiber decreased by 90% between 1880 and 1976. In addition to lower fiber content, refined wheat products also had fewer vitamins and other micronutrients. Machinery allowed the production of margarine and vegetable oils. Sugar imports and snacking increased in the Western world.

Obesity suddenly became very common in the upper classes of Europe and England toward the end of the 17th century and even more so in the 18th.

Weights also increased throughout populations of developed countries. For instance, if we look at U.S. men of average height between the ages of 30 to 34, average weights were 148 lb (66 kg) in 1863, but were up to 170 lb (77 kg) in 1963. Our current obesity epidemic didn't even start until around 1970.

Let's look at a few major U.S. diet changes from 1860 to 1975. Energy derived from protein rose from 12% to 14–15%. Energy from fat rose from 25 to 42% of calories. Energy from starches fell from 53 to 22%. Calories from sugar rose from 10 to 24%. Total carbohydrate calories fell from 63 to 46%.

It only takes a few decades to see major changes in a population's food consumption. For instance, U.S. per capita consumption of salad and cooking oils increased from 21.2 pounds (9.6 kg) per person in 1980 to 54.3 pounds (24 kg) per person in 2008 (USDA data). I refer to these oils as industrial seed oils, and they include soybean, corn, and sunflower oil. We're not entirely sure what effect these have on health. Some suspect they are related to obesity, heart disease, and other "diseases of civilization."

For instance, per capita soybean oil consumption in the U.S. increased over a thousand-fold between 1909 and 1999, to 7.4% of total calories. It's in many of our processed foods. Linoleic acid is a predominant omega-6 fatty acid in seed oils. Linoleic acid consumption increased by 200% in the last century.

Thanks to increasing omega-6 fatty acid consumption, the omega-6/omega-3 ratio increased from 5.4:1 to 9.6:1 between 1909 and 2009 (24).

The Industrial Revolution also introduced into our diets large amounts of man-made trans-fats, which are highly detrimental to cardiovascular health. Public outcry has lead to diminishing amounts of dietary trans-fats over the last decade.

Think about the typical Western or Standard American Diet (SAD) eaten by an adult these days (25). It provides an average of 2673 calories a day (not accounting for wastage of calories in restaurants; 2250 cals/day is probably a more accurate figure for actual consumption). Added sugars provide 459 of those calories, or 17% of the total. Grains provide 625 calories, or 23% of the total. Most of those sugars and grains are in processed, commercial foods. So added sugars and grains provide 40% of the total calories in the SAD. That's a huge change from the diet of our prehistoric ancestors. Remember, we need good insulin action to process these carbohydrates, which is a problem for diabetics and prediabetics. Anyone going from the SAD to pure paleo eating will be drastically reducing intake of added sugars and grains, our current major sources of carbohydrate. They'll be replacing them with foods that generally require less insulin for processing.

U.S. Department of Agriculture Fun Facts!
- A typical carbonated soda contains the equivalent of 10 tsp (50 ml) of table sugar.
- The typical U.S. adult eats 30 tsp (150 ml) daily of added sweeteners and sugars.
- U.S total grain product consumption was at record lows in the 1970s, at 138 pounds (63 kg) per person. By 2008, grain consumption was up by 45%, to 200 pounds (91 kg) per person.
- Total caloric sweetener consumption (by dry weight) was 110 pounds (50 kg) per person in the 1950s. By 2000, it was up 39% to 150 pounds (68 kg).

- Between 1970 and 2003, consumption of added fats and oils rose by 63%, from 53 to 85 pounds (24 to 39 kg). (How tasty would that be without starches and sugars? Not very.)
- In 2008, "added fat" calories in the U.S. adult diet were 641 (24% of total calories).

At his Whole Health Source blog, Dr. Stephan Guyenet and Jeremy Landen produced a graph of U.S. sugar consumption from 1822 to 2005. Dr. Guyenet wrote, "It's a remarkably straight line, increasing steadily from 6.3 pounds (2.9 kg) per person per year in 1822 to a maximum of 107.7 pounds (49 kg) per person per year in 1999. Wrap your brain around this: in 1822, we ate the amount of added sugar in one 12 ounce can of soda (360 ml) every five days, while today we eat that much sugar every seven hours."

Note that added sugars overwhelmingly supply only one nutrient: pure carbohydrate without vitamins, minerals, antioxidants, protein, fat, etc.

HEALTH EFFECTS OF THE AGRICULTURAL AND INDUSTRIAL REVOLUTIONS

Aren't people healthier now, thanks to the Agricultural and Industrial Revolutions? As a marker for health, we can look at life span and longevity. Humans started to see dramatic increases in longevity probably around 30,000 years ago, before the revolutions. Nevertheless, Kuipers, Joordens, and Muskiet note that average life expectancy after the start of the Agricultural Revolution 10,000 years ago fell from about 40 to around 20 years (26). Other researchers report that average height in the Nile River Valley at the time of the transition fell by 4 inches (10 cm). The Agricultural Revolution allowed for rapid expansion of human populations through more births, but those folks still didn't live very long. As before the revolution, infections and high infant/child mortality rates were devastating killers, dragging down average life spans. If you survived childhood, you had a shot at hitting 50 or 60.

At the dawn of the Industrial Revolution, life expectancy at birth was only 35–40 years, even in then-sophisticated cultures like Switzerland. Consider Thomas Jefferson, the principal author of the U.S. Declaration of Independence and the third U.S. president, who lived between 1743 and 1826 (he died on July 4, Independence Day). He and his wife Martha had six children; only two survived to adulthood, and only one past the age of 25. Martha died at age 33. This mortality picture was typical for the times.

Since 1800, life expectancy has doubled in industrialized countries, but it's mostly due to public health measures and economic prosperity. Other than smallpox vaccination, it wasn't until the mid-20th century that medical care advances contributed in a major way to longevity.

OVERVIEW

The following diseases may result from the mismatch of our Paleolithic genes and modern lifestyle (including diet): type 2 diabetes, high blood pressure, acne, osteoporosis, fertility problems (polycystic ovary syndrome), pregnancy complications (preeclampsia, gestational diabetes), some cancers (colon, breast, prostate), heart disease (such as coronary artery disease), major and postpartum depression, autism, schizophrenia, some neurodegenerative diseases (Parkinsons disease, Alzheimer's disease). Many of these are so-called "diseases of civilization."

OVERWEIGHT AND OBESITY

The Paleolithic diet is lower in total carbohydrate percentage-wise compared to the standard American diet: 30–35% versus 50–55% of calories. The higher consumption today, especially of highly processed refined carbohydrates, contributes to overweight and obesity, diabetes, gallbladder disease, heart disease, and possibly dementia.

Ian Spreadbury hypothesizes that carbohydrate density of modern foods may be the cause of obesity (27). Refined sugars and grains—types of acellular carbohydrates—are particularly bad offenders. These acellular carbs may alter our gut microorganisms, leading to systemic inflammation and leptin resistance, etc. Our Paleolithic ancestors had little access to acellular carbohydrates. Here's how Spreadbury explains acellular:

"Tubers, fruits, or functional plant parts such as leaves and stems store their carbohydrates in organelles as part of fiber-walled living cells. These are thought to remain largely intact during cooking, which instead mostly breaks cell-to-cell adhesion. This cellular storage appears to mandate a maximum density of around 23% non-fibrous carbohydrate by mass, the bulk of the cellular weight being made up of water. The acellular carbohydrates of flour, sugar, and processed plant-starch products are considerably more dense. Grains themselves are also highly dense, dry stores of starch designed for rapid macroscopic enzymic mobilization during germination. Whereas foods with living cells will have their low carbohydrate density "locked in" until their cell walls are breached by digestive processes, the chyme produced after consumption of acellular flour and sugar-based foods is thus suggested to have a higher carbohydrate concentration than almost anything the microbiota of the upper GI tract from mouth to small bowel would have encountered during our coevolution."

Added sugar provides 17% of total energy in modern societies, contributing to overweight, obesity, tooth decay, and diabetes.

Modern diets provide 15–20% of calories from protein, compared to 25–30% in the Paleolithic diet. To the extent that high protein consumption is satiating, lower consumption may cause over-eating of carbohydrates and fats, then overweight and obesity and all their associated medical conditions.

HEART DISEASE

I mentioned in the last chapter the much lower omega-6 to omega-3 fatty acid ratio in the Paleolithic diet. There's some evidence that today's high ratio may contribute to systemic inflammation and chronic disease, heart disease in particular. Today's ratio is quite high due to our consumption of industrial seed oils, such as those derived from soybeans, peanuts, corn, and safflower. And we don't eat enough cold-water fatty fish, which are major sources of omega-3 fatty acids. Two long-chain polyunsaturated fatty acids, EPA and DHA, are essential fatty acids. That means our bodies cannot make them. We have to get them from diet. DHA and EPA are also cardioprotective omega-3 fatty acids.

HIGH BLOOD PRESSURE

Most modern diets have much more sodium and much less potassium than the Paleolithic diet, perhaps contributing to high blood pressure, which in turn contributes to heart attacks, strokes, and possibly premature death. The higher magnesium content of the paleo diet may also help prevent high blood pressure.

GASTROINTESTINAL PROBLEMS

We eat much less fiber these days, contributing to constipation, hemorrhoids, and diverticulosis. Some experts believe low fiber consumption adversely effects development of palate bones, jaws, and tooth placement.

OSTEOPOROSIS

Our lower vitamin D levels these days may cause osteoporosis (thin fragile bones) and raise the risk of diabetes and cancer. Our prehistoric ancestors spent more time in the sun, allowing their bodies to make vitamin D.

TYPE 2 DIABETES

Robert Lustig and associates looked at sugar consumption and diabetes rates in 175 countries and found a strong link between sugar and type 2 diabetes (28). It's not proof of causation, just suggestive. From the scientific article abstract: "Duration and degree of sugar exposure correlated significantly with diabetes prevalence in a dose-dependent manner, while declines in sugar exposure correlated with significant subsequent declines in diabetes rates independently of other socioeconomic, dietary and obesity prevalence changes. Differences in sugar availability statistically explain variations in diabetes prevalence rates at a population level that are not explained by physical activity, overweight or obesity."

A major diet change from Stone Age to modern diets is a reduction in magnesium consumption. This could be one reason type 2 diabetes is a problem today. A 2013 article at *Diabetes Care* suggests that higher magnesium consumption in modern populations may protect against type 2 diabetes (29).

DENTAL PROBLEMS

Dentist John Sorrentino wrote at his blog in 2012 (30):
"The truth is that tooth decay is a relatively new phenomenon. Until the rise of agriculture roughly 10,000 years ago, THERE WAS NO TOOTH DECAY IN HUMANS. Let that sink in for a moment. Humanity is 2,500,000 years old. For the fist 2,490,000 years no one ever had a cavity. If we understand that tooth decay started when people started farming instead of hunting and gathering for a living clearly you realize that tooth decay is a disease or mismatch between what you are eating and what your body expects you to eat. If we examine the past as prologue it becomes clear that the path to proper health starts in the mouth and the answers are so simple that not only did a Cave Man do it. They perfected it."

To be fair and balanced, a research report from 2014 found a very high incidence of caries (cavities) in a Stone Age population living in what is now Morocco. The authors attributed the cavities to heavy consumption of acorns, which are rich in carbohydrates and sticky, to boot.

Orthodontist Mike Mew, BDS, MSc, made a presentation at the 2012 Ancestral Health Symposium titled "Craniofacial Dystrophy—Modern Melting Faces." Dr. Mew says 30% of folks in Western populations have crooked teeth and/or malocclusion, and the mainstream orthodontic community doesn't know why. But they've got expensive treatment for it! Dr. Mew thinks he knows the cause and he shared it at the symposium. The simple cure is "Teeth together. Lips together. Tongue on the roof of your mouth." And eat hard food that requires lots of chewing, like our ancestors did, ideally in childhood before age 9. Older people also benefit, he says.

NPR (National Public Radio) in February, 2013, ran an article called "Ancient Choppers Were Healthier Than Ours," by Audrey Carlsen (31). An excerpt:

> "Hunter-gatherers had really good teeth," says Alan Cooper, director of the Australian Centre for Ancient DNA. "[But] as soon as you get to farming populations, you see this massive change. Huge amounts of gum disease. And cavities start cropping up."

> And thousands of years later, we're still waging, and often losing, our war against oral disease.

> Our changing diets are largely to blame.

> In a study published in the latest Nature Genetics, Cooper and his research team looked at calcified plaque on ancient teeth

from 34 prehistoric human skeletons. What they found was that as our diets changed over time — shifting from meat, vegetables and nuts to carbohydrates and sugar — so too did the composition of bacteria in our mouths.

Not all oral bacteria are bad. In fact, many of these microbes help us by protecting against more dangerous pathogens.

Dentist Mark Burhenne wrote the following at Huffington Post—Canada (32):

It is generally well accepted that tooth decay, in the modern sense, is a relatively new phenomena. Until the rise of agriculture roughly 10,000 years ago, there was nearly no tooth decay in the human race. Cavities became endemic in the 17th century but became an epidemic in the middle of the 20th century (1950).

If we understand that tooth decay started when people started farming, rather than hunting and gathering, it's clear that tooth decay is the result of a mismatch between what we're eating and what our bodies are expecting us to eat based on how they evolved.

***

The recent changes in our lifestyle create a "mismatch" for the mouth, which evolved under vastly different environments than what our mouths are exposed to these days. Our mouths evolved to be chewing tough meats and fibrous vegetables. Sugar laden fruit was a rare and special treat for our paleolithic ancestors. Now, our diets are filled with heavily processed foods that take hardly any energy to chew — smoothies, coffees, and sodas high in sugar, white bread, and crackers to name just a few.

SHRINKING BRAINS

Since the end of the Stone Age, human brain size has been shrinking. That's not good, is it? Anthropologist John Hawks has noted that over the past 20,000 years, the average volume of the human male brain has decreased from 1,500 cubic centimeters to 1,350 cc, losing a chunk the size of a lemon. The female brain has shrunk proportionately. Anthropologists don't know why. Is it modern nutrition? The experts aren't sure what it means for our future. As for me, I think the answer is in Mike Judge's movie, "Idiocracy."

DEATH BY SUGAR

Sugar-sweetened beverages kill almost 200,000 worldwide annually, according to a Gitanjali Singh, Ph.D., a postdoctoral research fellow at the Harvard School of Public Health (33). How could that be? Sugar-sweetened beverages contribute to obesity, which in turn leads to diabetes, cardiovascular disease, and some cancers.

Reducing consumption of sugar-sweetened beverages was one of the major points in the American Heart Association's 2010 guidelines for reducing heart disease.

ELDERLY COGNITIVE IMPAIRMENT

Diets high in sugar and other carbohydrates raise the risk of elderly cognitive impairment, according to recent research by the Mayo Clinic (34). Mild cognitive impairment is often a precursor to incurable dementia. (Most authorities think dementia develops more often in people with diabetes, although some studies refute the linkage.) Researchers followed 940 patients with normal baseline cognitive functioning over the course of four years. Diet was assessed via questionnaire. Study participants were ages 70 to 89. As the years passed, 200 of them developed mild cognitive impairment. Compared with those eating the lowest amount of sugar, those eating the most sugar were 1.5 times more likely to develop cognitive impairment. Looking at total carbohydrate consumption, those eating at the highest levels of carbohydrate consumption were almost twice as likely to develop mild cognitive impairment. The scientists note that those eating lower on the carbohydrate continuum were eating more fats and proteins.

4
Diabetes: Causes and Abnormal Metabolism

Type 2 diabetes and prediabetes are epidemics now mostly because of excessive consumption of refined sugars and starches, and inadequate physical activity. Genetics and over-consumption of calories are among many other contributing or potentially causative factors.

WHAT'S WRONG WITH DIABETICS?

In type 1 diabetes, an autoimmune phenomenon causes the body to destroy it's own insulin-producing beta cells in the pancreas. Some cases have a hereditary cause; many cases are unexplainable. There's little we can do about the underlying disease-causing process in type 1 diabetes.

Thus far in the book I've broken down diabetes into types 1 and 2. In reality there are several more types. The only other one most readers might be interested in is called latent autoimmune diabetes of adulthood, or LADA.

I think of LADA as type 1 diabetes that starts in adulthood, although there are some differences from typical juvenile-onset type 1 diabetes.

Seven to 10% of apparent type 2 adult diabetics have LADA. It's caused by the body attacking its own pancreas beta cells and thereby impairing insulin production; in other words, it's an autoimmune thing, like in type 1 diabetes. Maybe it's genetic, maybe not. Here are some generalities (with exceptions, of course) about LADA, compared to typical type 2 diabetes:

- lower body mass index, often under 25
- age at onset under 50
- poorer response to dietary management
- poorer response to oral diabetic medications
- acute symptoms at time of diagnosis (e.g., weight loss, thirst, frequent urination, ketoacidosis, malaise)
- higher risk of developing diabetic ketoacidosis
- much more likely to need insulin

How is LADA diagnosed? First of all, the doctor has to consider the possibility, based on the clinical factors above. The autoimmune nature of the disease is reflected in islet-cell antibodies (ICA) and antibodies to glutamic acid decarboxylase (anti-GAD). These are testable in the blood. One of the two tests may be enough. If the disease is far enough along, blood levels of C-peptide will be low. C-peptide reflects the body's production of insulin.

Moving on to type 2 diabetes. The problem in type 2 diabetes and prediabetes is that the body cannot handle ingested carbohydrates in the normal fashion. In a way, dietary carbohydrates have become toxic instead of nourishing. This is a critical point, so let's take time to understand it.

NORMAL DIGESTION AND CARBOHYDRATE HANDLING

The major components of food are proteins, fats, and carbohydrates. We digest food either to get energy, or to use individual components of food in growth, maintenance, or repair of our own body parts.

We need some sugar (also called glucose) in our bloodstream at all times to supply us with immediate energy. "Energy" refers not only to a sense of muscular strength and vitality, but also to fuel for our brain, heart, and other automatic systems. Our brains especially need a reliable supply of bloodstream glucose. Red blood cells do, too. Most other tissues can and do utilize other energy sources, e.g., fat.

In a normal, healthy state, our blood contains very little sugar—about a teaspoon (5 ml) of glucose. (We have about one and a third gallons (5 liters) of blood circulating. A normal blood sugar of 100 mg/dl (5.6 mmol/l) equates to about a teaspoon of glucose in the bloodstream.)

Our bodies have elaborate natural mechanisms for keeping blood sugar normal. They work continuously, a combination of adding and removing sugar from the bloodstream to keep it in a healthy range (70 to 140 mg/dl, or 3.9 to 7.8 mmol/l). These homeostatic mechanisms are out of balance in people with diabetes and prediabetes.

By the way, glucose in the bloodstream is commonly referred to as "blood sugar," even though there are many other types of sugar other than glucose. In the U.S., blood sugar is measured in units of milligrams per deciliter (mg/dl), but other places measure in millimoles per liter (mmol/l).

When blood sugar levels start to rise in response to food, the healthy pancreas gland—its beta cells, specifically—secrete insulin into the bloodstream to keep sugar levels from rising too high. The insulin drives the excess sugar out of the blood, into our tissues. Once inside the tissues' cells, the glucose will be used as an immediate energy source or stored for later use. Excessive sugar is stored either as body fat or as glycogen in liver and muscle.

When we digest fats, we don't see much effect on blood sugar levels. That's because fat contains almost no carbohydrates. In fact, when fats are eat-en with high-carbohydrate foods, it tends to slow the rise and peak in blood sugar you would see if you had eaten the carbs alone.

DIETARY PROTEIN EFFECT ON BLOOD SUGAR

Ingested protein has the potential to raise blood sugar. When it happens, it's usually to a mild degree. As proteins are digested, our bodies can make sugar (glucose) out of the breakdown products. The process is called gluconeogenesis. The healthy pancreas releases at least some insulin to keep the blood sugar from going too high. The typical high-protein foods that might raise blood sugar are beef, chicken, pork, fish, and eggs, to name a few.

Is this effect of protein clinically significant? It's hard to say. For what it's worth, most dietitians and clinicians pay little attention to it as a source of hyperglycemia. That's because it's very difficult to determine in advance how much effect, if any, the protein will have. Variables that influence protein's ability to raise blood sugar include type 1 versus type 2 diabetes, the source of the protein and how much is eaten, how much insulin (if any) is still being made by the pancreas, the weight of the person eating, how much and what kind carbohydrate is also in the meal, how much fat is in the meal, the phase of the moon, etc.

On the other hand, diabetologist (and type 1 diabetic) Richard K. Bernstein, M.D., says dietary protein definitely has to be taken into account. Here are some of Dr. Bernstein's ideas pulled from the current edition of his book, *Diabetes Solution*:

- The liver (and the kidneys and intestines to a lesser extent) can convert protein to glucose, although it's a slow and inefficient process.
- Since the conversion process is slow and inefficient, diabetics don't see the high blood sugar spikes they would see from many ingested carbohydrates.
- For example, 3 ounces (85 g) of hamburger patty could be converted to 6.5 g of glucose under the right circumstances.
- Protein foods from animals (e.g., meat, fish, chicken, eggs) are about 20% protein by weight.
- Dr. B recommends keeping protein portions in a particular meal consistent day-to-day (for example 6 ounces with each lunch).
- He recommends at least 1–1.2 g of protein per kilogram of ideal body weight for non-athletic adults. That's more than the usual

recommended daily 0.8 g per kilogram for adults.

- The minimum protein he recommends for a 155-lb (70 kg) non-athletic adult is 11.7–14 ounces (370 g) daily.
- Growing children and athletes need more protein.
- On his eating plan, you choose the amount of high-protein food in a meal that would satisfy you, which might be 3 ounces (85 g) or 6–9 ounces (170–255 g).
- If you have gastroparesis, however, you should limit your evening meal protein to 2 ounces of eggs, cheese, fish, or ground meat, while eating more protein at the two earlier meals in the day.
- "In many respects—and going against the grain of a number of the medical establishment's accepted notions about diabetics and protein—protein will become the most important part of our diet if you are going to control blood sugars just as it was for our hunter-gatherer ancestors."

In case you're wondering, most folks in the developed world easily exceed the recommended daily protein amount of 0.8 grams per kilogram of ideal body weight. Getting enough protein is not usually a problem. Vegans or vegetarians may have to put some thought into it. None of my patients have ever been interested in calculating and monitoring their daily protein consumption.

To keep things simple, I tell my patients to eat a fair amount of protein-rich foods at each of three meals daily. Albert Einstein reportedly said, "Everything should be made as simple as possible, but not simpler." I agree with Dr. Bernstein that you should satisfy your hunger, whether that's three or nine ounces (85 or 255 g) of the aforementioned protein-rich foods. Women may be more comfortable at the lower end of the range, while men and highly athletic folks eat at the upper end. Consistency in the ounces from meal to meal and day to day may be important, especially if you're seeing wild fluctuations in blood sugars without obvious explanation.

DIETARY CARBHOHYDRATES HAVE THE MOST DRAMATIC EFFECT ON BLOOD SUGAR AND INSULIN REQUIRMENTS

In contrast to fats and proteins, carbohydrates in food cause significant—often dramatic—rises in blood sugar. The healthy pancreas, in turn, secretes higher amounts of insulin to prevent excessive elevation of blood glucose. Carbohydrates are easily digested and converted into blood sugar. The exception is fiber, which is indigestible and passes through us unchanged. (Actually, our gut bacteria can digest some of our ingested fiber, in turn producing short-chain fatty acids that we can absorb and use for energy. These are not major calorie sources for us, so forget I even told you.)

During the course of a day, the pancreas of a healthy person produces an average of 40 to 60 units of insulin. Half of that insulin is secreted in response to meals, the other half is steady state or "basal" insulin. The exact amount of insulin depends quite heavily on the amount and timing of carbohydrates eaten. Dietary protein has much less influence. A pancreas in a healthy person eating a very-low-carb diet will release substantially less than 50 units of insulin a day.

To summarize thus far: dietary carbs are the major source of blood sugar for most people eating "normally." Carbs are, in turn, the main cause for insulin release by the pancreas, to keep blood sugar levels in a safe, healthy range.

Hang on, because we're almost done with the basic science!

CARBOHYDRATE HANDLING IN DIABETES & PREDIABETES

Diabetics and prediabetics absorb carbohydrates and break them down into glucose just fine. Problem is, they can't clear the glucose out of the bloodstream normally. So blood sugar levels are of-ten in the elevated, poisonous range, leading to many of the complications of diabetes. Inadequate insulin action is the source of the problem.

Remember that insulin's primary function is to drive blood glucose out of the bloodstream, into our tissues, for use as immediate energy or stored energy (as fat or glycogen). In type 2 diabetes and prediabetes, this function of insulin is impaired.

Insulin also works on the liver to suppress the liver's production of glucose (gluconeogenesis).

In type 2 diabetes and prediabetes, the tissues have lost some of their sensitivity to insulin's action. This critical concept is called insulin resistance. Insulin still has some effect on the tissues, but not as much as it should. Different diabetics have different degrees of insulin resistance, and you can't tell by just looking.

Insulin resistance occurs in most cases of type 2 diabetes and prediabetes. So what causes the insulin resistance? In many cases it's related to overweight, physical inactivity, and genetics. A high-carbohydrate diet may contribute. A few cases are caused by drugs. Some cases are a mystery.

To overcome the body tissue's resistance to insulin's effect, the pancreas beta cells, if able, pump even more insulin into the bloodstream, a condition called hyperinsulinemia. Some scientists believe high insulin levels alone cause some of the damage associated with type 2 diabetes. While a healthy normal-weight person without diabetes needs about 50 units of insulin a day, an obese non-diabetic needs about twice that to keep blood sugars in check. Eventually, in those who develop type 2 diabetes or prediabetes, the pancreas can't keep up with the demand for more insulin to over-come insulin resistance. The pancreas beta cells get exhausted and start to "burn out." That's when blood sugars start to rise and diabetes and prediabetes are easily diagnosed. So, insulin resistance and high insulin production have been going on for years before diagnosis. By the time of type 2 diabetes diagnosis, 50% of beta cell function is lost.

Did you know that people who work at garbage dumps, sewage treatment plants, and cattle feedlots get used to the noxious fumes after a while? They aren't bothered by them as much as they were at first. Their noses are less sensitive to the fumes. You could call it fume resistance. In the same fashion, cells exposed to high insulin levels over time become resistant to insulin.

Remember that the basic problem in type 1 diabetes is that insulin production is minimal, if any, because an autoimmune process has destroyed the pancreas beta cells that make insulin. Type 1 diabetics usually don't have insulin resistance unless obese or have insulin antibodies that bind up and inhibit the action of injected insulin.

This explanation of diabetic physiology is an over-simplification, but most people aren't interested in further details and alternative explanations. If you are, see the Appendix for "Newer Theories on the Cause of Type 2 Diabetes."

EXTRA CREDIT FOR INQUISITIVE MINDS

You've learned that insulin's main action is to lower blood sugar by transporting it into the cells of various tissues. But that's not all insulin does. It also 1) impairs breakdown of glycogen into glucose, 2) stimulates glycogen formation, 3) inhibits formation of new glucose molecules by the body (gluconeogenesis), 4) promotes storage of triglycerides in fat cells (i.e., lipogenesis, fat accumulation), 5) promotes formation of fatty acids (triglyceride building blocks) by the liver, 6) inhibits breakdown of stored triglycerides, and 7) supports body protein production.

In his fascinating book, *Cheating Destiny: Living With Diabetes, America's Biggest Epidemic,* James Hirsch describes what happened to type 1 diabetics before insulin injections were available. Type 1 diabetics, remember, produce no insulin. Until Frederick Banting and Charles Best isolated and injected insulin in the early1920s, type 1 diabetes was a death sentence characterized not only by high blood sugars, but also extreme weight loss as muscle and fat tissue wasted away. The tissue wasting reflects insulin actions No.4, 5, 6, and 7 above.

Banting and Best worked at the University of Toronto in Canada. Their discovery of insulin is one of the greatest medical achievements of all time.

5
The Paleobetic Diet

Finally, what you've been waiting for. If you started the book here, please go back to the Introduction. It'll make a lot more sense.

A simple way to think of the Paleobetic Diet is that it's a low-carb diet minus the milk products, green beans, industrial seed oils, and artificial sweeteners.

In general, the modern Paleolithic diet is nutritionally adequate, if not superior to the Standard American Diet. I think it's superior. Two potential nutrient deficiencies of paleo diets are calcium and vitamin D, both of which are related to the lack of milk products. Milk is a great source of calcium, and milk products are often fortified with vitamin D. I'm not convinced that relatively low calcium consumption is a problem. Your body can make vitamin D if given adequate sun exposure. Both calcium and D are readily and cheaply available as supplements.

Obviously, I'm not your personal physician. If I were, I'd know your medical history, would have examined you recently, and would have reviewed recent lab results (blood work). Then I would know if it were safe for you to follow the program I outline here.

Since I don't know the details of your case, please note that the ideas and suggestions in this book are provided as general educational information only and should not be construed as medical advice or care. This information is meant to complement, not replace, any advice or information from your personal health professionals. All matters regarding your health require supervision by a personal physician or other appropriate health professional familiar with your current health status. Always consult your personal physician before making any dietary, medication, or exercise changes. Consult your dietitian and/or certified diabetes educator before making dietary changes. If any problems develop, always consult your personal physician. Only your physician can provide you medical advice. You should not follow this diet if you are a child, pregnant or lactating, have abnormal liver or kidney function, or have gout or a high uric acid blood level, because we don't have enough clinical information to ensure safety. If you take medications for high blood pressure or diabetes, they may need to be stopped or reduced by your personal physician.

You can familiarize your healthcare providers with the Paleobetic Diet by printing and giving them the brief outline available at the Paleo Diabetic website (54).

COMPONENTS

Nuts & seeds
Proteins
Vegetables
Fruits
Condiments & oils

DAILY CONSUMPTION

- 1–2 oz (30–60 g) nuts (primarily) or seeds
- Protein 3–8 oz (85–225 g) per meal (3 meals a day), or unlimited but consistent from day to day and meal to meal. Fish at least twice weekly.
- Two servings of low-carb vegetables (serving = 7 oz or 200 g) plus 1 or 2 servings of fruits (serving size below), starchy vegetables (serving size below), or more low-carbohydrate vegetables (serving = 7 oz or 200 g).
- Condiments and oils as needed for flavor and cooking.

Put together your own meals or get started with a week's worth of meals and special recipes in the next chapter. Keep track of your consumption, blood sugars, weight, and exercise with a daily log from the Paleo Diabetic website:
http://paleodiabetic.files.wordpress.com/2014/04/paleobetic-diet-daily-log.pdf
You'll also find a grocery shopping list:
http://paleodiabetic.files.wordpress.com/2014/04/paleobetic-diet-shopping-list.pdf
See chapter 10 (Daily Life With Paleo Eating) for additional help with meals.

NUTS AND SEEDS

Focus on walnuts, pecans, macadamia, cashews, almonds.

PROTEINS

Meat, fish, other seafood, eggs, poultry, offal, and wild game. Bacon is OK, but minimize it and other processed meats.

LOW-CARB VEGETABLES

GROUP A

Average digestible carbohydrate per 7 oz serving (200 g) is 5 g. The highest digestible carb counts are in scallions and jicama (8 g), and sweet peppers (7g).

Raw salad vegetables: lettuce, mushrooms, radishes, spinach, cucumber, tomato, scallions, parsley, jicama, arugula, kale, endive, radicchio, chard, sweet peppers, avocado, olives (pickled green or ripe black), pickles (dill or sour, not sweet or "bread and butter"), bok choy, escarole.

GROUP B

These average 8 g of digestible carbohydrate per 7 oz serving (200 g). Celeriac and onion are highest at 16 and 14 g, respectively. Weigh Group B veggies before cooking.

Solid or leafy vegetables, often cooked: artichoke hearts, broccoli, summer squash, zucchini, spaghetti squash, tomato, onion, cauliflower, eggplant,

Brussels sprouts, asparagus, bamboo shoots, okra, sauerkraut (canned), collard greens, beet greens, turnip greens, turnips, mustard greens, kale, chard, daikon radish, celeriac, kohlrabi, rhubarb, bok choy.

FRUITS

(Each serving has 7.5 grams of digestible carbohydrate.)

apple, a third of medium-sized one (54 g)
banana, one third (39 g)
peach, one half of medium (75 g)
strawberry halves, two thirds of a cup (75 g)
blueberries, one half cup (75 g)
raspberries, 1 cup (123 g)
blackberries, 1 cup (144 g)
cantaloupe, one half cup cubes (80 g)
honeydew, 1 cup of cubes (85 g)
date, medjool, one half date (12 g)
orange, navel, one half (70 g)
pear, a third of medium-sized one (60 g)
pomegranate, one fourth of 4" (10 cm) diameter fruit (70g)
tangerine, one half (44 g)
grapefruit, one half (61 g)
cherries, sweet, raw, a third of a cup (45 g)
grapes, a third of a cup (50 g)
raisins, seedless, 20 (9 g)
nectarine, medium, one half (70 g)
mango, slices, a third of a cup (55 g)
pineapple, raw chunks, a third of a cup (55g)
lime/lemon juice, raw, 2 limes or lemons (88 g)
watermelon, diced, two thirds of a cup (100 g)
plantain, raw, 1 oz or 28 g

STARCHY VEGETABLES

(Each serving has 7.5 grams of digestible carbohydrate.)

potato, white, raw, flesh and skin, one fourth of medium potato (53 g)
carrots, raw, strips or slices, three quarters of a cup (92 g)
sweet potato, raw, a third of 5 inch-long (13 cm) potato (45 g)
beets, canned, drained solids, three fourths of a cup slices (130 g)
cassava, raw, 3/4 oz or 21 g)
taro, raw, 1 oz or 28 g
parsnip, raw, 2 oz or 60 g
winter squash (e.g., acorn, butternut), raw, 1 cup of cubes (115 g)

CONDIMENTS AND OILS

Mustard, home-made vinaigrette, home-made mayonnaise (olive oil and egg yolk), cilantro, parsley, basil, rosemary, thyme, etc. Salt (minimal), pepper, vinegar. Oils: extra virgin olive, flax, avocado.

MISCELLANEOUS

1. Including scattered carbohydrates in condiments etc., this diet would total roughly 60 g of digestible carbs.
2. Try to limit breakfast digestible carbs to 10 g; limit lunch and dinner carbs to 20 g each.
3. To determine carbohydrate content of foods, use the USDA National Nutrient Database for Standard Reference (http://ndb.nal.usda.gov) or FitDay (http://fitday.com).

6
One Week of Meals + Special Recipes

The idea of trying a bunch of new recipes can be very intimidating. Will you be able to find the ingredients? How expensive are they? How time-consuming is the meal preparation? Will the final product be worth it?

Rest assured you don't have to make any of the recipes in this chapter to do the Paleobetic Diet. These recipes are just to give you some ideas for the future, or a way to get started tomorrow if you wish. Most people end up eating the same 10 or 12 meals over and over anyway. Nothing wrong with that if they're the right meals. So if the Paleobetic way of eating is new to you, you just need to come up with a couple handfuls of meals.

WHY BOTHER MAKING YOUR OWN MEALS?

I hate to be the one that has to tell you this, but if you want to control your diabetes, you need to know exactly what you're putting in your mouth. The best way to do that is to prepare your own meals. If you're over at a friend's house and are offered some home-made lasagna and a slice of apple pie, you won't have any idea how many carbohydrates are in them. And you won't have any idea how your blood sugar will respond.

The situation's a little better if you eat packaged food that has a nutrition facts label. You'll have a better idea how many digestible carb and protein grams and calories are in that food. Unfortunately, those labels are notoriously inaccurate. Restaurants that publish the nutritional analysis of their menu items have the same problem.

For example, if a serving of food allegedly has 50 grams of carbohydrate in it, the reality is that it may have 40 grams or it may have 60. That's a 20% variance both ways from 50. On the other hand, if your serving has 10 grams of carb, it may actually have between 8 and 12 grams. Still a 20% variance either way, but there's obviously a much larger absolute difference between 40 and 60 grams compared to 8 and 12. In terms of the effect on your blood sugar and diabetic drug dosages, you can disregard the difference between 8 and 12. Not so for the difference between 40 and 60.

According to diabetologist and type 1 diabetic Dr. Richard Bernstein, this is an example of his "laws of small numbers." Another way he phrases it is, "Big inputs make big mistakes. Small inputs make small mistakes." A real-world example would be adding salt to a pot of soup that needs some. You better add just small amounts at a time and re-taste frequently. When you make the mistake of adding too much salt right off the bat, you've ruined the soup. Not only do we have large margins of error in estimating carbs in food, we make big mistakes estimating the degree of absorption from insulin injections and the effectiveness of other diabetes drugs.

Minimize the inaccuracy of carb counting by preparing your own low-carb meals. This chapter will help get you started. On the other hand, if you have experience with food and cooking, you may be able to review the basic tenets of the Paleobetic Diet and just run with. Here they are again:

DAILY CONSUMPTION

- 1–2 oz (30–60 g) nuts (primarily) or seeds
- Protein 3–8 oz (85–335 g) per meal (3 meals a day), or unlimited but consistent from day to day and meal to meal. Fish at least twice weekly.
- Two servings of low-carb vegetables (serving = 7 oz or 200 g) plus 1 or 2 servings of fruits (serving size below), starchy vegetables (serving size below), or more low-carbohydrate vegetables (serving = 7 oz or 200 g).
- Condiments and oils as needed for flavor and cooking.

See chapter 10 (Daily Living With Paleo Eating) for information on grocery shopping, additional recipe sources, recommended cookbooks and cooking instruction books, how to handle sweet cravings, and weight loss tips.

ABOUT THE RECIPES

Most of these are easy to prepare and can be done in 30 minutes or less. No specialized equipment is needed. If I mention a "prominent feature" in the nutritional analysis, it typically means that the specified nutrient provides at least 40 % of the Recommended Dietary Allowance (RDA) or Adequate Intake (AI) for a non-pregnant adult eating 2,000 calories a day.

Many of the recipes yield three or four servings, so you can have leftovers for subsequent days and not have to start from scratch. We value your time.

None of the ingredients should be hard to find in common supermarkets. You can choose organic fruits and vegetables, grass-fed pastured beef, wild-caught salmon, and free-range happy chickens at your own prerogative.

If a meal calls for a small apple for dessert but they're out of season and too expensive, just substitute a cheaper in-season fruit that has the same amount of digestible carbohydrate. (Digestible carb grams = total carb grams minus fiber grams.) For example, a small apple with skin has 17 g of digestible carbs, while a cup of sweet raw cherries has 18 g. Close enough. It took me only three minutes to figure that out at SELFNutritionData: http://nutritiondata.self.com.

We like avocados at the Parker compound. If you don't, and a meal calls for eating avocado slices, you can substitute one-half or three-quarter ounces (15–20 g) of nuts for half a California avocado. The carb grams are similar.

You can print nearly all of these recipes from the Paleo Diabetic website: http://paleodiabetic.com.

If you're still hungry after eating the designated serving size, or if you think you're just not getting enough calories, eat more of the food item in the meal that is lowest in carbohydrate and highest in protein of fat. Protein in particular tends to be satiating. The protein foods are things like beef, chicken, fish, and eggs. Nuts are high in fat content, but it would be better for your blood sugar levels to eat 200 calories of fat than 200 calories of carbohydrate.

The daily calorie counts for the meals here are in the range of 1,800 to 2,000. That may be too much for some (women?) and too few for others (men or athletes?). Adjust accordingly. If you're losing weight but don't have the extra fat to lose, eat more! Eat more protein and fat calories. If you need to lose fat weight, don't try for losing more than a pound or pound-and-a-half per week (2–3 kg). If you're losing too fast, eat more. See chapter 10 (Daily Living With Paleo Eating) for weight-loss tips.

DAY 1

Breakfast: Brian's Berry Breakfast

4.5 oz (127 g) fresh strawberries, diced into small pieces
2 oz (58 g) walnuts, crumbled by hand

Mix ingredients together in a bowl and enjoy eating with a spoon while your tablemates eat their cold cereal with milk.

Servings: 1

Nutritional Analysis:
76% fat
16% carbohydrate
8% protein
410 calories
17 carb grams
6.2 g fiber
10.9 g digestible carb
2 mg sodium
436 mg potassium
Prominent features: Rich in vitamin C, copper, manganese

Lunch: Tossed Tuna Salad and Almonds

This is an easy lunch or dinner. For a different flavor and twice the calcium, you could substitute canned sardines for the tuna, but I've never tried it.

lettuce, romaine, 3.5 oz (100 g), in bite-size chunks
onion, chopped, 1.5 oz (42 g)
tomatoes, chunked, 5.5 oz (150 g)
tuna, canned, albacore/white, packed in water
    (drain and discard the fluid), 5-oz can (140 g)
olive oil, extra virgin, 1.5 tbsp (22 ml)
vinegar, balsamic, 1/2 tbsp (7.5 ml)
salt and pepper to taste (not counted in nutritional
    analysis below)
almonds, 1.5 oz (45 g)
lemon juice (optional)

In a 3-quart (3-liter) bowl, put lettuce, onion, tomatoes, and tuna (3.25 oz or 90 g at this point). Add olive oil, balsamic vinegar, and salt and pepper to taste. Mix well with a fork. For extra flavor, consider adding a few squirts of fresh lemon juice. This is a neat trick if you're trying to avoid salt. Enjoy almonds separately, before, during, or after salad.

Servings: 1

Nutritional Analysis:
58% fat
12% carbohydrate
30% protein
711 calories
22.3 g carb
9.4 g fiber
12.9 digestible carb
670 mg sodium
1,392 mg potassium
Prominent features: Good source of protein, vitamin B12, vitamin E, copper, niacin, phosphorus, and selenium

Dinner: Lemon-Pepper Chicken, Vegetable Medley, and Salad

The ingredients here are for two servings. Your grocery store may sell a large bag of vegetables called "vegetable medley" that has equal parts broccoli, cauliflower, and carrots.

chicken breasts, boneless, skinless, frozen, 16 oz
    (450 g)
commercial lemon pepper seasoning (choose one
    with low sodium and the fewest non-paleo
    ingredients like sugar)
broccoli, fresh, raw, 4.5 oz (130 g), bite-size pieces
cauliflower, fresh, raw, 4.5 oz (130 g), bite-size
    pieces
carrots, fresh, raw, 4.5 oz (130 g), peeled and sliced
    into bite-size pieces
commercial low-sodium vegetable seasoning (e.g.,

Weber Roasted Garlic and Herb)
lettuce, Romaine, 6 oz (170 g), bite-size chunks
tomatoes, raw, 6 oz (170 g), bite-size chunks
cucumber, raw, 4 oz (115 g), peeled and sliced
celery, raw, 4 oz (115 g), sliced
sunflower seed kernels, dry roasted, without salt, 1
    oz (30 g)
bacon bits (aka crumbled bacon), 2 tbsp (15 g)
olive oil, extra virgin, 5 tbsp (75 ml)
vinegar, 1 tbsp (15 ml) (your choice of red wine,
white wine, balsamic, or apple cider vinegar)
garlic, raw, 1 clove, sliced very thinly
salt and pepper to taste (not counted in the
    nutritional analysis below)
lemon, fresh (optional)

Start on the chicken first. Sauté the breasts in a
non-stick pan over medium heat. You don't need to
thaw it beforehand. While cooking, sprinkle with the
lemon pepper seasoning. If the breasts are thick,
you may want to "butterfly" them with a knife when
half done, to speed up the cooking process. If you
over-cook, the meat will be tougher. It should be
done in roughly 10–15 minutes. While the chicken
is cooking, get to work on your other items.

Cook the vegetables thusly. Put the broccoli, cauliflower, and carrots in a microwave-safe dish, add
about four fl oz (120 ml) of water, and microwave
(covered) on high for four minutes. If you don't have
a cover, just use a water-moistened paper towel.
While they cook, heat 2 tbsp (30 ml) of the olive oil
in a medium-sized pan over low heat, with the garlic, for a couple minutes to release the garlic flavor.
Drain the water off the microwaved vegetables, then
sauté them in the olive oil pan over medium-high
heat for a couple minutes, stirring frequently. Add
your commercial vegetable seasoning when you

start sautéing or at any point thereafter, even at the table.

Finally the salad. In a large bowl, place the lettuce, tomatoes, sunflower seeds, cucumber, celery, bacon bits, 3 tbsp (45 ml) olive oil, and vinegar. Mix thoroughly.

You might enjoy a few squirts of fresh lemon juice on the vegetables or salad just before eating.

Servings: 2

Nutritional Analysis Per Serving:
55% fat
12% carbohydrate
32% protein
800 calories
27 g carbohydrate
11 g fiber
16 g digestible carb
970 mg sodium (not counting any you add, such as in commercial seasonings)
1830 mg potassium
Prominent features: Generous amounts of protein, vitamin A, Vitamin B6, vitamin C, vitamin E, niacin, pantothenic acid, phosphorus, and selenium

DAY 2

Breakfast: Fried Eggs, Cantaloupe, and Macadamia Nuts

eggs, large, 3
olive oil, 2 tsp (10 ml)
salt to taste (1 dash)
pepper to taste
cantaloupe or honeydew melon, fresh, peeled and

slivered, 6 oz (170 g)
macadamia nuts, roasted, 1 oz (30 g)

Spread olive oil in bottom of pan, then fry eggs, adding salt and pepper as desired. Enjoy macadamia nuts as you cook. Finish your meal and refresh your palate with the melon.

Servings: 1

Nutritional Analysis:
72% fat
13% carbohydrate
16% protein
555 calories
18.7 g carbohydrates
3.8 g fiber
14.9 g digestible carbohydrate
468 mg sodium
758 mg potassium
Prominent features: Rich in protein, vitamin A, vitamin B12, vitamin C, iron, pantothenic acid, riboflavin, and selenium

Lunch: Chili With a Side of Cucumber

chili, 1.5 cups (360 ml) (See Special Recipes at the
    end of the chapter)
cucumber, fresh, 7-inch (18 cm or 200 g), peeled
    and sliced

Servings: 1

Nutritional Analysis:
68% fat
10% carbohydrate
21% protein
780 calories

23 g carbohydrate
5 g fiber
18 g digestible carbohydrate
1,384 mg sodium
1,429 mg potassium
Prominent features: Good source of protein, vitamin B6, vitamin B12, copper, iron, niacin, selenium, thiamine, and zinc

Dinner: Baked Trout, Vegetable Medley, and an Apple

Trout are one of the cold-water fatty fishes loaded with the omega-3 fatty acids that are so good for our hearts and brains. Paleolithic man ate much more omega-3 and less omega-6 fatty acids than modern man. Eating cold-water fatty fish is a great way to get back to that ancestral balance. This recipe serves two.

trout, fresh filets, 16 oz (450 g)
broccoli, raw, fresh, 4.5 oz (130 g), bite-size chunks
cauliflower, raw, fresh 4.5 oz (130 g), bite-size chunks
carrots, raw, fresh, 4.5 0z (130 g), bite-size chunks
olive oil, extra virgin, 7 tbsp (100 ml)
garlic, raw, 4 cloves (12 g), thinly sliced or finely diced
parsley, raw, 1.5 tbsp (6 g), chopped
basil, fresh, 4 leaves (1.5 g), chopped
lemon juice, 3/4 fl oz (22 ml)
salt, 1/2 tsp (2.5 ml)
black pepper, 1 tsp (5 ml)
commercial low-sodium vegetable seasoning of your choice
apples (2), fresh, medium size, (2.75-inch or 7-cm diameter)

First, make a marinade. In a glass or plastic bowl, mix 5 tbsp (75 ml) of the olive oil, 3 of the diced garlic cloves (9 g), parsley, salt, pepper, lemon juice, and basil.

Place the trout in a medium sized (8 or 9-inch or 21-cm diameter) glass baking dish, then cover with the marinade. Let sit in the refrigerator for 1–2 hours, turning occasionally.

Preheat oven to 375 degrees F (190 degrees C). Pull the fish dish out of the refrigerator when you start the preheat process. Cover the glass dish with aluminum foil, then bake in oven for 20–40 minutes. This is a judgment call. When done, it should flake apart readily with a fork. This cooking method works well for trout, salmon, cod, tilapia, and perhaps others. Consider squeezing fresh lemon juice on the cooked fish for extra zing.

Start on the vegetables about ten minutes after the fish go in the oven. Put the broccoli, cauliflower, and carrots in a microwave-safe dish, add about four fl oz (120 ml) of water, and microwave (covered) on high for four minutes. If you don't have a cover, just use a water-moistened paper towel. While they cook, heat 2 tbsp (30 ml) of the olive oil in a medium-sized pan over medium heat (with one clove of diced garlic) for a couple minutes to release the garlic flavor. Drain the water off the microwaved vegetables, then sauté them in the olive oil pan for a couple minutes, stirring frequently. Add your commercial vegetable seasoning when you start sautéing or at any point thereafter, even at the table. Enjoy the apple for desert.

Servings: 2

Nutritional Analysis Per Serving:

59% fat
16% carbohydrate
25% protein
840 calories
36 g carbohydrate
9 g fiber
27 g digestible carbohydrate
790 mg sodium (plus your vegetable seasoning amount)
1,620 mg potassium
Prominent features: Generous amounts of omega-3 fatty acids, protein, vitamin A, vitamin B6, vitamin B12, vitamin C, vitamin E, copper, iron, manganese, niacin, pantothenic acid, phosphorus, riboflavin, and thiamine

DAY 3

Breakfast: Mexican Eggs and Avocado Slices

If you don't want to make a batch of the pico de gallo, substitute an amount of commercial picante sauce that provides no more than three grams of digestible carbohydrate. "Digestible carbohydrate" is the total carb grams of a serving, minus the fiber grams.

eggs, three large
tomato, fresh, 2 oz (60 g)
onion, fresh 3/4 oz (20 g)
jalapeño pepper, fresh, 1/4 of a pepper
cilantro, fresh, 3-4 sprigs chopped finely to supply 1
    tbsp (15 ml)
olive oil, 2 tsp (10 ml)
California avocado, 1 whole (these are the dark
    green or black avocados, usually 4 x 2.5 inches

or 10 x 5 cm)
salt, to taste (1/4 tsp?)
black pepper to taste (1/4 tsp?)

Make the pico de gallo first. Finely chop and mix together the tomato, onion, jalapeño pepper, cilantro, and salt and pepper to taste.

Peel and slice the avocado. Salt and pepper to taste. Fry the eggs in an olive oil-coated pan. Salt and pepper to taste. When done, transfer to a plate and spoon the pico de gallo onto the eggs. Enjoy with avocado slices on the side.

Servings: 1

Nutritional Analysis:
72% fat
13% carbohydrate
15% protein
592 calories
20.4 g carbohydrate
12.8 g fiber
7.6 g digestible carbohydrate
810 mg sodium (if you use a total of 1/4 tsp)
1,237 mg potassium
Prominent features: Good sources of fiber, vitamin B6, vitamin B12, vitamin E, copper, iron, pantothenic aci, riboflavin, and selenium

Lunch: Cabbage Soup, Salad, and an Apple

Hearty Cabbage Soup, 2 cups (See Special Recipes
    at the end of the chapter)
baby spinach, 2 oz (60 g)
lettuce, romaine, 2 oz (60 g), bite-size pieces
tomatoes, chunked, 3 oz (85 g)
cucumbers, peeled and sliced, 2 oz (60 g)

olive oil, extra virgin, 2 tbsp (30 ml)
vinegar, 2 tsp (10 ml)
salt and pepper to taste (not counted in nutritional
    analysis below)
apple, medium (2.75-inch or 7-cm diameter)
lemon juice (optional)

See Special Recipes at the end of this chapter for
Hearty Cabbage Soup.

Salad: In a bowl, place the lettuce, spinach, tomato
chunks, sliced cucumber, and finally, the olive oil
and vinegar. Mix thoroughly. Salt and pepper to
taste. If you're avoiding salt, consider substituting a
few squirts of fresh lemon juice.
Enjoy the apple for desert.

Servings: 1

Nutritional Analysis:
61% fat
26% carbohydrate
13% protein
550 calories
38.7 g carb
10.3 g fiber
28.4 g digestible carb
1,252 mg sodium (plus any you add)
1,328 mg potassium
Prominent features: Good source of vitamin A, vitamin B12, vitamin C, vitamin E, copper, iron, and
zinc

**Dinner: Flank Steak, Guacamole, Cucumber, and an Or-
ange**

Flank steak is sometimes called jiffy steak. If you
can't find it, use skirt steak. In any case, the beef
steak used in this is never over an inch (2.54 cm)

thick. These are not particularly tender cuts, so have your butcher run the steak through a mechanical tenderizer. This recipe serves two.

flank steak, mechanically tenderized, 24 oz (680 g)
 (this cooks down to 14 oz or 400 g)
California avocados, 2 (about 5.5 oz or 155 g each,
 measuring 2.5 x 3.5 inches or 6.4 x 9 cm)
tomato, fresh, 1.5 oz (43 g), finely diced
onion, fresh, 0.5 oz (14 g), finely diced
salt, a pinch or 1/16 tsp
black pepper to taste
low-sodium steak seasoning (I use McCormick Grill
 Mates Montreal Steak Seasoning, which is
 coarse salt (1/4 tsp has 180 mg sodium), spices
 including black and red peppers, garlic,
 sunflower oil, natural flavor, extractives of
 paprika) (or just use salt and pepper to taste)
oranges, 2 medium sized (2.6 inch or 6.5 cm
 diameter)
cucumber, fresh, 1 large (8 inches or 20 cm long),
 peeled and sliced

First, start the steak frying in a non-stick pan over medium heat. Sprinkle with steak seasoning or salt and pepper. Cook until done to your liking.

While the steak's cooking, make your guacamole. Slice the avocados in half and remove the seeds, then scoop out the flesh into a bowl and mash it with a fork until pasty yet still a little chunky. Blend in the tomato, onion, and a pinch of salt. It's done. Enjoy the cucumber as a side dish and the orange for desert.

Servings: 2 servings of 7-oz steak (200 g), 8 tbsp (120 ml) guacamole, half a cucumber, and an orange

Nutritional Analysis Per Serving:
46% fat
16% carbohydrate
38% protein
730 calories
31.5 g carbohydrate
13.7 g fiber
18 g digestible carbohydrate
968 mg sodium
2,065 mg potassium
Prominent features: Rich in fiber, protein, vitamin B6, vitamin B12, vitamin C, copper, iron, niacin, pantothenic acid, phosphorus, riboflavin, selenium, and zinc

DAY 4

Breakfast: Bacon, Eggs, and Honeydew Melon

3 large eggs
3 strips of bacon, standard thin slices
Salt and pepper to taste
1/2 cup raw honeydew melon, cubed

Fry the bacon over medium or medium-high heat. If there's too much grease leftover in the pan after cooking, poor out what you don't want, for later use or drizzle over your dog's dry kibble food. Leave a little grease in the pan so your eggs don't stick. Then fry your eggs over medium heat. Enjoy with raw honeydew, which will cleanse your palate after eating bacon.

Servings: 1

Nutritional Analysis per Serving:
63 % fat
10 % carbohydrate

26 % protein
319 calories
9 carbohydrate grams
1 fiber grams
8 digestible carbohydrate grams
845 mg sodium
423 mg potassium
Prominent features: High in B12, riboflavin, selenium, protein, pantothenic acid, and phosphorus. Although this is low in calories, it's adequately satiating because of the rich protein and fat content. The calorie count will be higher by 50 if you eat all the bacon grease.

Lunch: Spaghetti Squash Spaghetti

Yeah, I know. Spaghetti's not paleo. But this one is because it's not grain-based.

With the Paleobetic Diet, I strive to limit mealtime digestible carbohydrates to 20 g or less. This meal has 29 g and the calories are on the low end (408) for larger and more active folks. What gives?

Making a wholesale switch from the Standard American Diet to the paleo diet can be difficult for some under the best of circumstances. For those used to eating carb-heavy pasta, I thought it might be comforting to offer something similar but with a lower carb count. Hence, spaghetti squash spaghetti. The tomatoes in the sauce are an additional source of blood glucose-elevating carbohydrates. So I've tried to minimize them by creating a meat-heavy sauce. Nevertheless, a reasonable portion size (two cups) tipped me over the 20 gram carb limit. One cup of the spaghetti squash has 8 g of digestible carb and 60 calories. In contrast, a cup of cooked wheat-based spaghetti pasta has 38 grams of digestible carbohydrate and 200 calories. I think you'll find the two cups of spaghetti squash filling and satisfying. If that's not enough calories for you, munch on some leftover high-protein food such as chicken or steak.

3/4 cup (240 ml) low-carb spaghetti sauce (see
    Special Recipes at the end of this chapter)
2 cups (480 ml) cooked spaghetti squash as in
    Special Recipes

Put the spaghetti squash on a plate and cover with the sauce. Enjoy.

Number of Servings: 1

Nutritional Analysis:
52% fat
33% carbohydrate
15% protein
408 calories
36 g carbohydrate
7 g fiber
29 g digestible carbohydrate
1,398 mg sodium
1,201 mg potassium
Prominent features: Rich in B12, copper, iron, niacin, thiamine, B6

Dinner: Naked Chicken Fajitas, Walnuts, and a Pear

My earliest recollection of fajitas is from Austin, Texas, in 1981. I had just moved there from Oklahoma City to start my internship and residency in Internal Medicine at Brackenridge Hospital. Back then fajitas were made with skirt steak, the diaphragm of a cow or steer. It was considered a cheap low-quality cut of meat. You can also make fajitas with chicken. The contents of a fajita are wrapped in a tortilla usually made with flour. Since we're a paleo crowd, we'll skip the tortilla. Use lettuce as a wrapper if you wish.

I wonder if the El Azteca Restaurant is still in business in Austin. Best Mexican food I ever had. I think it was on 6th Street or so, about 3/4 mile east of I-35. Good times.

By the way, the j in fajita is pronounced "h." Accent on second syllable. "Fuh-HEET-uh."

Today we're using chicken and making four servings. If you use skirt steak instead, the nutritional analysis will be very similar; I wouldn't worry about the differences.

I have different fajita recipe using skirt steak marinated in commercial Zesty Italian Dressing in the refrigerator overnight or for at least four hours. Grill it over coals outside. Yum! I don't recall whether I added lemon juice to the marinade or squirted it on the meat just before serving. You would just cook the onions and peppers on a pan on the stove as above, with salt and pepper to taste. Garnish with a margarita and I'll make you an honorary Texan.

1 lb (454 kg) chicken breast, raw, boneless and skinless, cut in strips about 1/4-inch wide (you can often buy it this way)
7 oz onion, raw, cut in long crescent shapes about a 1/4-inch wide (0.6 cm)
6 oz (170 g) bell pepper, raw, cut in long strips roughly a 1/4-inch wide (these are also called sweet peppers; a combination of the red and green ones is eye-pleasing)
2 tbsp (30 ml) olive oil
5 or 6 oz (155 g) tomato, raw, cut in long strips

1 tsp (5 ml) salt
1/2 tsp (2.5 ml) pepper
1/2 tsp (2.5 ml) chili powder
1 tsp (5 ml) parsley flakes
1/2 tsp (2.5 ml) oregano leaves
1 pinch of cumin
1/2 tsp (2.5 ml) paprika
Optional: You could replace all these spices with a
    1-oz (28 g) pack of Lawry's Chicken Fajitas
    Spices & Seasoning. The sodium and potassium
    values below would be different.
1/3 cup (80 ml) water
16 oz (454 g) lettuce (e.g., iceberg, romaine, or bibb)
4 oz (113 g) walnuts
4 pears, small (about 1/3 lb or 150 g each))

Instructions:

Add the onions, peppers, and 1 tbsp (15 ml) olive oil
to a 12-inch (30 cm) skillet and cook at medium-
high heat until tender, stirring occasionally. This'll
take about 10 minutes. Set the skillet contents
aside.

The vegetables reduce volume by half while cooking
In the same pan, add 1 tbsp (15 ml) olive oil and the
chicken and cook at medium to medium-high heat,
stirring frequently, until chicken is thoroughly
cooked. For me, this cooked quicker than the vegetables. But don't overcook or the chicken will get
tough. Then add the water and all the spices. Bring
to a boil while stirring occasionally, then simmer on
low heat a few minutes. This is your fajita filling.

My original plan was to make "fajita wraps," wrap-
ping the cooked fajitas into a large leaf of iceberg
lettuce. This was pretty messy, especially since I
love the sauce in the bottom of the pan. I tried two
leafs as a base: still messy. Finally I just made a bed

of lettuce (4 oz) and loaded the fajita concoction right on top. Eat with a knife and fork. Mess gone. Try a different lettuce? Skip the lettuce entirely and you can reduce digestible carb count in each serving by 2 grams.

Enjoy the walnuts and pear with your meal.

Number of servings: 4

Serving size: A cup (240 ml) of the fajita mixture, 4 oz (113 g) lettuce, 1 oz (28 g) walnuts, 1 small pear. One cup makes two lettuce wraps.

Nutritional Analysis Per Serving:
48% fat
26% carbohydrate
26% protein
Calories: 514
37 g carbohydrate
10 g fiber
27 g digestible carbohydrate (25 g if you skip the lettuce)
928 mg sodium
904 mg potassium
Prominent features: Rich in protein, vitamin B6, vitamin B12, vitamin C, copper, iron, manganese, niacin, phosphorus, and selenium

DAY 5

Breakfast: BLT Avocado Wrap and Pecans

As I've written before, bacon isn't a pure paleo food. Cavemen didn't eat it. It's too highly processed. You could make your own if you want. But store-bought bacon is convenient and no doubt better for you—at least if you have diabetes—than many of our traditional breakfast foods like cereal with milk, pancakes, instant oatmeal, bagels, or donuts. Those could shoot your blood sugar up to the moon.

Some studies link processed meats with cardiovascular disease and cancer, other studies don't. If you want to be cautious with your health, don't go hogwild with bacon or other processed meats like hot dogs, bologna, and liverwurst.

Avocados come in hundreds of varieties. In the U.S., we mainly have California avocados (aka Hass) and Florida avocados. Californians are by far the market leader. They reign at the Parker Compound.

California avocados are the smaller dark green lumpy-skinned ones. Florida avocados are larger, smoother-skinned, and lighter green.

Did you know avocados are fruits, not vegetables?

1 California (Hass) avocado, raw, medium size (about 4 x 2.5 inches or 10 x 6 cm), peeled and seeded, cut into long strips
6 bacon strips, medium thickness
4 oz (115 g) lettuce (e.g., iceberg, romaine, bibb, or broad-leaf lettuce you prefer)
4 oz (115 g) tomato, raw (this is about one-and-a-half roma tomatoes or one medium regular tomato), cut into long strips
1 oz (30 g) pecans (option: substitute your favorite tree nut except for cashews—too many carbs)

Fry your bacon in a skillet over medium to medium-high heat. Next you're gong to build two wraps. Lay out about 2 oz (60 g) of lettuce and load it with three bacon strips, half your tomato, and half your avocado. Fold or wrap lettuce edges together and enjoy. Repeat with remaining ingredients. The pecans are for dessert.

Number of Servings: 1 (that's 2 wraps plus nuts)

Nutritional Analysis:
74% fat
12% carbohydrate
14% protein
720 calories
24 g carbohydrate
15 g fiber
9 g digestible carbohydrate
1137 mg sodium
1507 mg potassium
Prominent features: Good source of fiber, sodium, protein, vitamin B6, niacin, thiamine, pantothenic acid, copper, manganese, phosphorus, and selenium

Lunch: Apple-Pecan-Blueberry Lunch Bowl

2.5 oz (70 g) apple, diced ("red delicious" variety
    works well) (this is half a medium-sized apple)
2.5 oz (70 g) pecans, crumbled into small pieces
2.5 oz (70 g) raw blueberries

Mix all together in a bowl, then enjoy. I know a lotta you bros will just eat all the components individually, but try the mix once for new flavors.

Servings: 1

Nutritional Analysis:
76% fat
20% carb
4% protein
570 calories

30 g carbohydrate
10 g fiber
20 g digestible carb
1.4 mg sodium
421 mg potassium
Prominent features: Good source of copper, manganese, and thiamine. Inadequate protein to get you through the day, but you'll make up for it at breakfast or dinner.

Dinner: Beef Soup, Asparagus, and Blackberries

The entree is a cross between stew and soup; stoup, if you will.

2 lb (0.9 kg) stew meat, lean, bite-sized chunks
    (tenderized by the butcher if able)
1 garlic clove, finely minced
6 sprigs cilantro, de-stemmed, whole leaves
2 oz (58 g) sweet onion, diced (1/2 of a small onion)
1/4 of a medium-size green bell pepper, de-seeded,
    diced (medium bell pepper weighs about 5.5 oz
    or 155 g)
8 oz (227 g) canned tomato sauce
2.5 cups (590 ml) water
1.25 tsp (6.2 ml) table salt
freshly ground black pepper to taste (1/4 tsp or 1.2
    ml?)
16 oz (454 g) fresh raw asparagus, no larger in
    diameter than your little finger, with any dry or
    woody stalk cut off and discarded
1.5 tbsp extra virgin olive oil
7.5 oz (213 g) raw blackberries

Stoup first. In a frying pan or electric skillet, place the stew meat, cilantro, garlic, bell pepper, onion, and cook over medium heat (350° F or 177° C) until the meat is done. Then add the tomato sauce, two cups of the water, one tsp of the salt, and pepper to taste. Simmer for two hours, then add a half cup water to replace evaporation loss.

Now the asparagus. Preheat oven to 400° F or 204° C. Place asparagus on a cooking sheet covered with foil, brush the asparagus with the olive oil, then lightly salt (1/4 tsp?) and pepper to taste. (If you don't mind cleaning up, just use a baking dish without the foil.) Roast in oven for 8–15 minutes; thicker asparagus takes longer. It's hard to tell when it's done just by looking; if it's still hard, it's not done. Enjoy the berries for desert.

Servings: 3 (one serving is 1.5 cups (355 ml) of soup, a third of the asparagus (5 oz or140 g), and 2.5 oz (70 g) berries)

Nutritional Analysis:
40 % fat
12 % carbohydrate
48 % protein
590 calories
19 g carbohydrate
8.5 g fiber
10.5 g digestible carb
1,557 mg sodium
1,778 mg potassium
Prominent features: High in protein, vitamin B6, vitamin B12, copper, iron, niacin, phosphorus, selenium, and zinc

DAY 6

Breakfast: Turkey Tomato Bowl and Macadamia Nuts

This is what I did with some of our leftover Thanksgiving turkey. If you don't have leftover turkey, I bet leftover chicken or steak would be fine substitutes. Heck, I'm tempted to try it with salmon or canned tuna or chicken. In addition to the flavor, what I like about this meal is that it's crazy quick.

The recipe calls for balsamic vinaigrette. I was lazy when I made this so I just used a commercial salad dressing rather than making my own vinaigrette. The bottle of famous name-brand vinaigrette dressing boasted "with extra virgin olive oil." Here were the top ingredients, in order: *water*, balsamic vinegar, soybean oil and extra virgin olive oil, sugar, salt, spices, etc. So the oil could have been soybean oil (from a legume—the horror!!!) with just one drop of extra virgin olive oil for all I know. The serving size was two tbsp (30 ml), providing three grams of carbohydrate (all sugar) and only 60 calories.

I don't know any home cooks who add water to vinaigrettes. They are essentially oil and vinegar (in a ratio of 3:1) and spices. The ones I make have quite a bit more than 60 calories per two tbsp (30 ml); more like 220 cals. All of the oils you would use have about 120 calories per tbsp, nearly all from fat. If you make this recipe with home-made vinaigrette, add 150 calories to the nutritional analysis below. It won't affect the carb count. You'll find a vinaigrette recipe in the Special Recipes section at the end of this chapter.

Note that of the common vinegars, balsamic has the most carbohydrates—some vinegars have zero. If you use typical amounts of balsamic vinaigrette, you shouldn't need to worry about the carbohydrates unless perhaps you're on a strict ketogenic diet and limited to 20–30 grams of carb daily.

6 oz (170 g) cooked turkey chunks, light meat (or 8 oz (225 g) if you're starting raw and planning to

cook it)
5 oz (140 g) raw tomato (2 small roma tomatoes, for
    example), cut into chunks
2 tbsp (30 ml) balsamic vinaigrette
black pepper to taste
1 oz (30 g) roasted macadamia nuts

Toss the turkey and tomato chunks in a bowl,
splash on the vinaigrette, then microwave for 60–80
seconds. Pepper as desired. Drink the leftover juice
right out of the bowl. Enjoy with macadamia nuts
for dessert and you've got a full meal.

Servings: 1

Nutritional Analysis:
58% fat
7% carbohydrate
35% protein
620 calories (870 if you used home-made
    vinaigrette)
11.5 g carbohydrate
3.7 g fiber
8 g digestible carbohydrate
743 mg sodium
877 mg potassium
Prominent features: High in protein, vitamin B6,
iron, manganese, niacin, phosphorus, selenium,
and zinc

Lunch: Shrimp Salad and Strawberries

This was inspired by a shrimp/spinach salad I like
at Applebee's, a chain restaurant. But here I eschew
the sweetness of their sauce and delete the bacon
bits.

If fresh strawberries aren't in season, substitute an equal amount of cantaloupe or honeydew melon, or 14 sweet raw cherries, or 1/2 cup (78 g or 120 ml) of blueberries. The carb count stays the same.

5 oz (140 g) raw shrimp tails, shell removed
1 tbsp (15 ml) parsley, finely chopped (we used the curly variety)
1 garlic clove, finely chopped
1/4 tsp (1.2 ml) pepper
1/4 tsp (1.2 ml) salt
1 tbsp (15 ml) extra virgin olive oil
1/2 tsp (2.5 ml) extra virgin olive oil
2 oz (57 g) baby spinach (or romaine lettuce or mix of both)
2 oz (57 g) cucumber, peeled and diced
2 tbsp AMD vinaigrette (or commercial dressing with 2 or fewer digestible carbohydrate grams per 2 tbsp or 30 ml) (Find the AMD vinaigrette in the Special Recipes section at the end of this chapter)
2 and 3/8 oz or 1/2 cup (67 g or 120 ml) fresh strawberries, sliced (3–4 medium berries)

Make the vinaigrette first so the components have some time to synergize.

Next, you'll sauté the shrimp. In a bowl, combine the raw shrimp, parsley, 1/2 tsp (2.5 ml) olive oil, garlic, salt, and pepper, then mix thoroughly to evenly coat the shrimp. Alternatively, you could do that mixing in a plastic baggie (bisphenol-A!). Add 1 tbsp (15 ml) olive oil to a frying pan and cook the shrimp over medium heat until opaque, stirring continuously. When done, it will be patchy pink and white. It only takes about three minutes.

On a large plate, lay out a bed of spinach or lettuce, over which you'll scatter the cucumber and cooked shrimp, then the vinaigrette.

Enjoy the fruit for desert.

Servings: 1

Nutritional Analysis:
63% fat
14% carbohydrate
23% protein
590 calories
23 g carbohydrate
6 g fiber
17 g digestible carbohydrate
1,349 mg sodium
904 mg potassium
Prominent features: Rich in protein, vitamin B12, A, C, E, copper, iron, manganese, and selenium

Dinner: Brian Burger With Bacon Brussels Sprouts, Tomato, and Pistachios

Here's another meal recipe from my stepson. This makes three servings. You'll want to make the Bacon Brussels Sprouts to serve with other meals, so I've provided an additional nutritional analysis for those alone.

13 oz (370 g) ground beef, 85% lean
1/2 tbsp (7.5 ml) Tessemae's All Natural Dressing-Marinade-Dip "Southwest Ranch," or A1 Steak Sauce or balsamic vinaigrette or AMD vinaigrette (See Special Recipes) (Brian recommends the Tessemae's Dressing)
1.7 oz (50 g) onion, diced coarse or fine
1 garlic clove, diced
1/8 tsp (0.5 ml) paprika

1–2 pinches of salt (pinch = 1/16 tsp) pepper to taste (a pinch or two?)

1/4 tsp (1.2 ml) dried rosemary, crumbled or crushed

1/2 large egg, whisked to blend white and yolk

3 oz (85 g) lettuce

1 lb (450 g) Brussels sprouts (cut and discard bases if desired, probably doesn't matter), shredded

8 oz (225 g) bacon (6.5 regular (not thick) 8-inch strips), diced

3 tbsp (45 ml) water

1.5 large tomatoes, sliced

4.5 oz pistachio nuts

First cook the bacon in a pan over medium–high heat until done. Don't discard the grease.

Next do your Brussels sprouts prep (shredding). It will take a few minutes to shred it with a knife. Set those aside.

Start on the burgers now. Place the ground beef in a bowl then add your chosen sauce or vinaigrette, onion, egg, garlic, paprika, rosemary, salt, and pepper. Mix thoroughly by hand. Divide the mess into three patties of equal size. Fry or grill over medium heat until done, about 10 minutes.

As soon as the burgers are plopped on the heat, start steaming the shredded sprouts thusly. Take a pan with a lid, add 3 tbsp (45 ml) of the bacon grease and the 3 tbsp of water, then heat that up for a minute or two over medium to high heat. Then throw in the shredded sprouts, salt and pepper to taste (probably unnecessary), and cover with a lid. Immediately reduce heat to medium and cook for 4–6 minutes. The sprouts will soften up as they cook. Gently shake the pot every minute while steaming to prevent contents from sticking to the pan. If necessary, remove the lid and stir while cooking, but this may increase your cooking time since you release hot steam whenever you remove the lid. When the sprouts are done, remove from heat and add the remaining bacon and bacon grease, then blend.

Serve the burger on a bed of lettuce (1 oz or 30 g). Enjoy tomato and pistachios on the side. Serving sizes are below.

Number of Servings: 3 (one burger patty, 1 oz (30 g) lettuce, 1 cup (240 ml) of sprouts, 1/2 tomato or a third of all the slices, 1.5 oz (40 g) pistachio nuts)

Nutritional Analysis per Serving:
58% fat
17% carbohydrate
25% protein
740 calories
32 g carbohydrate
12 g fiber
20 g digestible carbohydrate
827 mg sodium
1,802 mg potassium
Prominent features: Rich in fiber, protein, vitamin B6, B12, C, copper, iron, manganese, niacin, pantothenic acid, phosphorus, riboflavin, selenium, thiamine, and zinc

Nutritional Analysis for Bacon Brussels Sprouts: (1 cup, no added salt):
47% fat
28% carbohydrate
26% protein
180 calories
14 g carbohydrate
6 g fiber
8 g digestible carbohydrate

530 mg sodium
709 mg potassium
Prominent features: Mucho vitamin C.

DAY 7

Breakfast: Steak, Avocado, Olives, and Tomato

This was super-easy to put together because I used leftover steak. But I'll assume you're cooking your steak fresh. We bought ours as thinly sliced round steak, about a 1/4-inch thick (0.6 cm). Some places might refer to this as a "minute steak" because it cooks so quickly. Minute steak also refers to a piece of beef, usually the round, that's been pounded flat, about a 1/4-inch thick. Even if you start with raw meat, you can prepare today's recipe in 10 minutes.

4 oz (113 g) cooked thin round steak (start with 5 oz raw)
1 California (Hass) avocado, standard size (4.5 oz or 127 g), peeled, pitted, and chunked
14 black olives, pitted, medium size (Paleo purist alert: probably highly processed)
1 tomato, medium-size (medium size or 2.5-inch diameter (6,4 cm), or a large roma tomato), cut into wedges
Salt and pepper to taste, or use commercial steak seasoning such as Montreal Steak Seasoning by McCormick (a favorite at the Parker Compound)

Sprinkle your steak with seasoning then cook over medium or medium-high heat in a skillet, about a minute on each side. Or heat your leftover steak in the microwave. If you overcook, it will be tough.

Place all ingredients artfully on a plate and enjoy.

Servings: 1

Nutritional Analysis:
60% fat
12% carbohydrate
28% protein
600 calories
20 g carbohydrate
12 g fiber
8 g digestible carbohydrate
587 mg sodium
1530 mg potassium
Prominent features: Lots of protein, vitamin B6, vitamin B12, copper, iron, niacin, pantothenic acid, phosphorus, selenium, and zinc

Lunch: Sunny's Super Salad

This huge salad is a full meal. It fills a 10-inch plate (25 cm). Since it contains five vegetables, you should feel virtuous eating it. Who says the paleo diet is all about meat?

8 oz (230 g) raw chicken breast tenderloin (it cooks down to 5 oz)
1/4 cup (60 ml) canned mandarin orange wedges (6-7 wedges) (if you can only find these packed in syrup or light syrup, add 3 g to the digestible carb count below)
1/4 tsp (1.2 ml) lemon pepper seasoning
4 oz (110 g) hearts of romaine lettuce
1 oz (30 g) baby spinach
2.5 oz (1/4 cucumber or 70 g) cucumber, peeled and sliced into discs
2 oz (60 g) California avocado, peeled and seeded, cut into wedges (1/2 of standard-sized avocado)
3 oz (85 g) fresh tomato (a typical roma or small tomato)

1 oz (30 g) walnuts
6 tbsp (90 ml) extra virgin olive oil
2 tbsp (30 ml) vinegar (we used balsamic)
1/4 tsp (1.2 ml) salt
1/4 tsp (1.2 ml) fresh ground black pepper
1/4 tsp (1.2 ml) crushed dried rosemary

First cook the chicken breast over medium heat in a skillet. If you think the meat will stick to the pan, add a smidgen (1/2 tsp or 2.5 ml) of olive oil to the pan. Don't overcook or the meat will get tough. It'll take five or 10 minutes.

While that's cooking, prepare your vinaigrette. In a jar with a lid, place the olive oil, vinegar, salt, pepper, and rosemary, then shake vigorously for 20 seconds. Not 21 or you'll ruin it. You're done.

If you use a commercial vinaigrette instead, use one that has no more than 2 g of carbohydrate per 2 tbsp. You may have trouble finding that since so many of the commercial guys add sugar.

Place the lettuce and spinach on a plate then add the cucumber, avocado, tomato, cooked chicken, walnuts, and mandarin orange wedges on top. Drizzle two or three tbsp (30–45 ml) of the vinaigrette over it (nutritional analysis assumes three). Enjoy.

Servings: 1

(Actually, you'll have enough vinaigrette left over for one or two more salads or vegetable servings. Save it in the refrigerator.)

Servings: 1

Nutritional Analysis:
57 % fat

12 % carbohydrate
31 % protein
710 calories
25 g carbohydrate
10 g fiber
15 g digestible carb
990 mg sodium
1,570 mg potassium
Prominent features: Rich in protein, vitamin A, vitamin B6, vitamin C, copper, iron, manganese, magnesium, pantothenic acid, selenium, and phosphorus

Dinner: Baked Glazed Salmon and Herbed Spaghetti Squash

This is a paleo-friendly modification of a meal in my low-carb Mediterranean diet book. It makes two servings.

16 oz (450 g) salmon filets
4.5 garlic cloves
7 tsp (34.5 ml) extra virgin olive oil
1.5 fl oz (45 ml) white wine
4.5 tsp (22 ml) mustard
4 tbsp (60 ml) vinegar, either cider or white wine
    (balsamic vinegar would add 6 g of carbohydrate
    to each serving)
2 tsp (10 ml) honey
1.5 tbsp (15 ml) fresh chopped oregano (or 1 tsp (5
    ml) of dried organo)
2 cups cooked spaghetti squash from Special
    Recipes at the end of this chapter
2 tbsp fresh parsley, chopped
0.5 tsp (2.5 ml) salt
1/4 tsp (1.2 ml) black pepper, or to taste

Start on the herbed squash first since it may take 30 to 70 minutes to cook unless you use the microwave method. To two cups of the cooked squash, add 4 tsp (20 ml) of the olive oil, all the fresh chopped parsley, a half clove of minced garlic, 1/3 tsp (1.6 ml) of the salt, and 1/8 tsp (0.6 ml) of black pepper, then mix thoroughly. The herbed squash is done. It could be difficult to time perfectly with the fish even if you have two ovens. But it's tasty whether warm, room temperature, or cold. If you want it warm but it's cooled down before the fish is ready, just microwave it briefly.

Onward to the fish. Preheat the oven to 400° F (200° C). Line a baking sheet or pan (8" or 20 cm) with aluminum foil. Lightly salt and pepper the fish in the lined pan, with the skin side down.

Now the glaze. Sauté four cloves of minced garlic with 1 tbsp (15 ml) of olive oil in a small saucepan over medium heat for about three minutes, until it's soft. Then add and mix the white wine, mustard, vinegar, honey, and 1/8 tsp (0.625 ml) of salt. Simmer uncovered over low or medium heat until slightly thickened, about there minutes. Remove glaze from heat and spoon about half of it into a separate container for later use.

Drizzle and brush the salmon in the pan with the glaze left in the saucepan. Sprinkle the oregano on top.

Bake the fish in the oven for about 10–13 minutes, or until it flakes easily with a fork. Cooking time depends on your oven and thickness of the fish. Overcooking the fish will toughen it and dry it out. When done, use a turner to transfer the fish to plates, leaving the skin on the foil if able. Drizzle the glaze from the separate container over the filets with a spoon, or brush it on. Don't use the unwashed brush you used earlier on the raw fish.

Servings: 2

Nutritional Analysis:
50% fat
13% carbohydrate
37% protein
600 calories
21 g carbohydrate
3 g fiber
18 g digestible carbohydrate
1,150 mg sodium
1,277 mg potassium
Prominent features: Rich in protein, vitamin B6,
vitamin B12, niacin, pantothenic acid, phosphorus,
and selenium

SPECIAL RECIPES

Chili

If you're making chili, you might as well make a
batch you can dip into over several days. It only gets
better with time (up to a point!). This recipe provides
eight servings of 1-cup (240 ml) each.

ground beef (80% lean, 20% fat), raw, 20 oz (570 g)
pork Italian sausage, raw, 20 oz (570 g)
onion, 1 large, diced
tomatoes, diced, canned, 14.5 oz (410 g)
tomato paste, 4 oz (115 g)
garlic, 5 cloves, peeled and thinly sliced
salt, 1/2 tsp (2.5 ml)
allspice, ground, 1/4 tsp (1.2 ml)
chili powder, 2 tbsp (30 ml)
cinnamon, ground 1/2 tbsp (7.5 ml)
cayenne pepper, ground, 1/4 tsp, (1.2 ml)
water, 1 cup (240 ml)

Cut the Italian sausage into small pieces. Sauté the sausage, ground beef, onion, and garlic in a large pot. Don't just brown the meat; cook it thoroughly. When done, drain off the fat if desired (but why waste those good calories?). Add the remainder of ingredients, bring to a boil, then simmer for about an hour. Add additional water if the chili looks too thick.

Servings: 8 servings of 1-cup (240 ml) each.

Nutritional Analysis Per Serving:
70% fat (if not drained off after cooking)
9% carbohydrate
21% protein
475 calories
11.4 g carbohydrate
2.3 g fiber
9.1 g digestible carbohydrate
860 mg sodium
722 mg potassium

Hearty Cabbage Soup

This is easy but takes a while to cook. This batch provides four servings of 2 cups (475 ml) each. Incidentally, if you're a constipated, a bowl or two of cabbage soup may get things moving.

water, 4 quarts (3.8 L)
parsley, fresh, to taste (3 or 4 sprigs)
stew meat (beef), raw, 8 oz (230 g)
pepper, to taste (1/4 tsp or 1.2 ml)
salt, to taste (1.5 tsp or 8.4 mL) (don't use this
    much if on a low-sodium diet)
tomato sauce, canned, 4 fl oz (120 ml)
carrot, raw, large (4.5 oz or 130 g), peeled and sliced

into 1/4-inch (1/2-cm) thick discs
cabbage, green, raw, 1/2 of a small one (whole one
   weighs about 2 lb or 900 g), rinsed, cored, then
   sliced into quarters or smaller
fresh lemon (optional)

Add raw meat to the water in a large pot and boil
gently for 30 minutes. Then add tomato sauce, carrot, salt, pepper, parsley, and cabbage. Bring to boil
over medium heat and them simmer for 45 minutes.
If it's too bland for you, add a squeeze of fresh lemon. Or as a last resort, add some beef bouillon cube
or powder.

Servings: 4 servings of 2 cups each (475 ml).

Nutritional Analysis Per Serving:
46% fat
23% carbohydrate
31% protein
200 calories
12 g carbohydrate
3 g fiber
9 g digestible carb
1,200 mg sodium
495 mg potassium

Pico De Gallo

This is a condiment for eggs, meat, or guacamole,
for example.

tomatoes, fresh, 7 oz (200 g), chopped very finely
onion, fresh, 2 oz (56 g), chopped very finely
jalapeno pepper, fresh, 1 (14 g), chopped very finely
   (discard stem first)
cilantro, fresh, 10–15 sprigs chopped to yield 3–4

tbsp (2 g)
salt to taste (a couple pinches or 2/16 tsp)

If you prefer less spicy heat, use less jalapeno and discard the seeds. Combine all ingredients. Eat at room temperature, chilled, or heated at medium heat in a saucepan (about 5 minutes, until jalapenos lose their intense green color).

Servings: 3 servings of 1/2 cup (120 ml) each.

Nutritional Analysis Per Serving:
8% fat
81% carbohydrates
11% protein
80 calories
4.5 g carbohydrate
1.2 g fiber
3.3 g digestible carbohydrate
104 mg sodium (2 pinches of added salt)
216mg potassium

Spaghetti Squash

It's hard to give up pasta. Many diabetics who keep eating it notice that their blood sugar levels spike too high when they eat pasta. What's too high? In general, I'd say over 150 mg/dl (8.33 mmol/l) measured one hour after a meal, or over 130 mg/dl (7.22 mmol/l) two hours after the meal. Other experts disagree and propose other numbers.

An alternative to spaghetti pasta that shouldn't raise blood glucose levels as high is spaghetti squash. It's all about the carbohydrates. A cup of cooked spaghetti squash has 10 g of carb; a cup of cooked spaghetti has 43 g. The fiber grams are about the same, 2 g.

Spaghetti squash is a classic low-carb vegetable. If you've never tried it, you should. As vegetables go, it's one of the largest, heaviest, and most interesting to prepare. Easy, too. The spaghetti squash season is autumn and winter in the northern hemisphere. Purchasing in spring and summer may be iffy.

In my part of the world, supermarket spaghetti squashes weigh between two and five pounds. We cooked a three-pounder (1.4 kg) that yielded five cups; a five-pounder (2.3 kg) gave us 12 cups. A serving size is one, maybe two cups. What you don't eat immediately stays fresh in the refrigerator for at least several days. Re-heat by microwaving or stir-frying.

Like pasta and potatoes, the squash by itself is bland. It's a great substrate for sauces or seasonings.

There are a couple ways to cook spaghetti squash. First, the traditional oven baking method. Preheat the oven to 375° F or 190° C. Very carefully slice the squash in half lengthwise. Spoon out and discard the guts (seeds and membranes like a pumpkin; it even smells like a pumpkin). Put the halves flat-side down in a pan, then add a half inch (1.3 cm) of water to the pan. Cover with foil and bake until the outer shell (rind) is fairly easily pierced with a paring knife. This will be about 45 minutes for a two-pound squash (0.9 kg); 90 minutes for a four-plus pounder (2.3+ kg). Then turn them over, re-cover with foil, and cook 15 minutes more, until very tender. Remove from the oven and allow them to cool for a few minutes. Then use a fork to pull the strands away from the rind.

Other cooks simplify the process and just place the squash halves flat-side down on a baking sheet and cook for 30-60 minutes. Some leave the seeds in while cooking and spoon them out just before the stranding step.

The other way of cooking is microwaving. First microwave the whole squash for one minute. Then cut in half lengthwise and remove the seeds and membranes. Take a microwave-safe baking dish and put water in it to a depth of a half inch or 1 cm. Place the squash in the dish, cut side down, and cook in the microwave for about 12 minutes or until tender to a fork. Carefully remove the squash (it's hot!) and use a fork to remove the pasta-like strands.

Now what?

You got options.

Our first experiment was with low-carb spaghetti sauce (see the next recipe).

Next we took three cups squash (710 ml) and mixed in 2 tbsp (30 ml) extra virgin olive oil, 2.5 tbsp (37 ml) chopped parsley, 1/2 tsp (2.5 ml) minced fresh garlic, 1/2 tsp (2.5 ml) salt, and 1/8 tsp (0.6 ml) black pepper.

Finally, we took a cup (240 ml) of the squash and added minced celery (4 inches or 10 cm of stalk), 3 minced black olives, 5/8 oz (18 g) of minced sweet (bell) pepper, 1/2 clove of minced garlic, salt (a dash), and pepper to taste.

These last two options I consider side dishes. They have eight to 10 grams of digestible carb per cup (240 ml). By the way, they taste good either cold or warm. They would go well with a number of entrees, such as steak or salmon.

I've read that this squash is good with pesto, or just with salt and (non-paleo) butter.

One cup of cooked spaghetti squash has around 60 calories (sources vary from 40 to 80), 10 g of carbohydrate, 2 g of fiber, 8 g of digestible carb, 4 g of fat (predominantly MUFA), minimal protein, and a fair amount of vitamins A, niacin, B6, and C. Plus 8% of your RDA for manganese.

Low-Carb Spaghetti Sauce

My wife is Italian so we eat a lot of spaghetti. A definitely non-paleo ingredient below is Truvia, a sweetener that's a combination of stevia and erythritol. Stevia is supposedly "natural." I don't know where erythritol, a sugar alcohol, comes from. The purpose of a sweetener is to counteract the tartness or bitterness of the tomatoes. Honey would probably serve this purpose, but I've never tried it in this recipe. If you use the honey or table sugar option below, it will increase the digestible carb count in each cup by three grams. Whatever your favorite noncaloric sweetener, use the equivalent of two tablespoons of table sugar (sucrose). You can also just leave the sweetener out if you're a very-low-carb paleo purist.

1 lb (454 g) sweet Italian sausage, removed from
    casing
3/4 lb (340 g kg) lean ground beef (lean = up to 10%
    fat by weight)
1/2 cup (118 ml) onion, minced
2 cloves garlic, crushed
1 can crushed tomatoes (28 oz or 793 g)

2 cans tomato paste (total of 12 oz or 340 g)
2 cans tomato sauce (total of 16 oz or 454 g)
1/2 cup water (118 ml)
2 tsp (10 ml) Truvia (combo of stevia and erythritol);
   optional substitutes are table sugar (2 tbsp or
   30 ml) or honey (1.5 tbsp or 22 ml), or leave out
   sweetener
1.5 tsp (7.4 ml) dried basil leaves
1/2 tsp (2.5 ml) fennel seeds
1 tsp (5 ml) Italian seasoning
1/4 tbsp (3.7 ml) salt
1/4 tsp (1.2 ml) ground black pepper
4 tbsp (60 ml) fresh parsley, chopped

Put the sausage, ground beef, onion, and garlic in a pan and cook over medium heat until well browned. Drain off the excess liquid fat if that's your preference (not mine). You'll probably have to transfer that mix to a pot, then add all remaining ingredients and simmer on low heat for two or three hours. You may find the flavor even better tomorrow. If it gets too thick, just add water.

To avoid carbohydrate toxicity—high blood sugar— eat this over spaghetti squash rather than pasta. Small or inactive folks may find a half cup of sauce over one cup of cooked squash is a reasonable serving (about 250 calories). I prefer to double those portions, making it a whole meal.

Sometimes I just eat this sauce straight. But I'm weird. A cup of sauce with some veggies or fruit is a meal for me. One of my blog readers likes spaghetti sauce over cooked zucchini that has been cut lengthwise in long strips.

Number of Servings: 9 (1-cup each)

Nutritional Analysis: (assumes you retained all fat)

55% fat
23% carbohydrate
22% protein
345 calories
21 g carbohydrate
4 g fiber
17 g digestible carbohydrate
985 mg sodium
1,117 mg potassium

Prominent features: Rich in vitamin B12, iron, copper, niacin, sodium, and selenium

Steamed Brussels Sprouts

This is a variation of the bacon Brussels sprouts in the Brian Burger meal on Day 6, which used raw bacon that you cooked to produce bacon bits. The bacon grease was also used. To make it a little more convenient, here I've substituted off-the-shelf real bacon bits instead of frying my own bacon. I traded olive oil for the bacon grease. The two versions taste very similar.

1 lb (454 g) Brussels sprouts, raw, shredded (slice
     off and discard the bases first)
4 tbsp (60 ml) extra virgin olive oil
5 tbsp (75 ml or 35 g real bacon bits or crumbles
     (e.g., by Hormel or Oscar Mayer)
2 garlic cloves, minced (optional)
1/8 (0.6 ml) tsp salt
1/4 tsp (1.2 ml) ground black pepper
3 tbsp (45 ml) water

You'll be steaming this in a pan with a lid. Put the garlic and olive oil in a pan and cook over medium-high heat for a few minutes to release the flavor of the garlic. Add the water to the pan and let it warm up for a half a minute or so on medium-high heat. Then add the shredded sprouts and cover with the lid. After a minute on this medium-high heat, turn it down to medium. The sprouts will have to cook for only 4–6 minutes. Every minute, shake the pan to keep contents from sticking. You might need to remove the lid and stir with a spoon once, but that lets out your steam and may prolong cooking time. The sprouts are soft when done. Then remove from heat, add the bacon bits, salt, and pepper, then mix thoroughly.

I'd like to experiment with this by leaving out the bacon and using various spices instead.

Number of Servings: 3 (1 cup or 240 ml each)

Nutritional Analysis per Serving:
71% fat
19% carbohydrate
10% protein
270 calories
14 g carbohydrate
6 g fiber
8 g digestible carbohydrate
328 mg sodium
646 mg potassium
Prominent feature: High in vitamin C (over 100% of your RDA)

AMD Vinaigrette

Classic vinaigrettes are very low in carbohydrate content. On the other hand, many commercial salad dressings are "enhanced" with added sugar, which you don't need if you have diabetes. On top of that, most are made with industrial seed oils, like soybean, so they're not paleo-approved. Avoid the unnecessary carbs and industrial seed oils by making your own vinaigrettes.

You may be able to find a commercially prepared vinaigrette in the salad dressing section of the supermarket. If so, be sure the predominant oil is olive oil (not very common) and that a serving (usually two tbsp or 30 ml) has no more than 2 g of carb.

The basic vinaigrette recipe is three parts olive oil to one part vinegar. We prefer extra virgin olive oil. Add salt, pepper, and other spices at your whim. Blend with a whisk, or put all ingredients in a jar with a lid and shake it. If you're watching your carbohydrate consumption, choose red wine or white wine vinegar before balsamic. I suppose you could use apple cider vinegar, too. Any vinaigrette you make like this will have negligible carb content.

This following recipe was in my 2007 book, *The Advanced Mediterranean Diet*; hence, "AMD vinaigrette."

Try this on salads, fresh vegetables, or as a marinade for chicken, fish, or beef. If using as a marinade, keep the entree/marinade combo in the refrigerator for 4–24 hours. Seasoned vinaigrettes taste even better if you let them sit for several hours after preparation. Mix a batch and keep it in the refrigerator—it should be good for at least five days. The olive oil will solidify, so take it out and set at room temperature for an hour before using. Shake before using.

I'll warn you, this is pretty spicy. If you prefer less tang, either use less of the vinaigrette, or reduce these particular ingredients by half: lemon juice, salt, pepper, paprika, and mustard.

2 garlic cloves (6 g), minced
juice from 1 lemon (40–50 ml)
2/3 cup (160 ml) extra virgin oil olive
4 tbsp (16 g or 60 ml) fresh parsley, finely chopped
1 tsp (5 ml) salt
1 tsp (5 ml) yellow mustard
1 tsp (5 ml) paprika
4 tbsp (60 ml) red wine or apple cider vinegar

In a bowl, combine all ingredients and whisk together. Alternatively, you can put all ingredients in a jar with a lid and shake vigorously—my preferred method. Let sit at room temperature for an hour, for flavors to meld.

Number of Servings: 6 servings of 2 tbsp (30 ml).

Nutritional Analysis per Serving:
98% fat
2% carbohydrate
0% protein
220 calories
1.4 g carbohydrate
0.3 g fiber
1 g digestible carbohydrate
400 mg sodium
41 mg potassium

Of course even were the narrative totally BS, I'd
venture most folks' paleo diets are exceedingly
healthful given the emphasis on actual cooking.

—Yoni Freedhoff, M.D.

7

Hypoglycemia: Recognition and Management

The Paleobetic Diet may provide fewer carbohydrates than you're used to eating. For instance, the typical American diet supplies 250 to 300 grams of digestible carbohydrate daily. In contrast, the Paleobetic Diet delivers in the range of 45 to 80 grams of carbohydrate. Carbohydrate-restricted diets are often so effective at controlling blood sugars that low blood sugar (hypoglycemia) becomes a serious risk for some diabetics. It's rarely a problem in prediabetes. But people with diabetes using particular drugs could develop life-threatening hypoglycemia, particularly when switching to a low-carb style of eating.

CARBOHYDRATES AND BLOOD SUGAR

Never forget that carbohydrate consumption has a major effect on blood sugar (glucose) levels—often causing a rise—in many people with diabetes and prediabetes. Most folks with diabetes are taking medications to lower their glucose levels.

Remember that the main components of food (called macronutrients) are proteins, fats, and carbohydrates. Common carbohydrate sources are:

- grains
- fruits
- starchy vegetables (e.g., potatoes, corn, peas, beans)
- milk products
- candy
- sweetened beverages
- other added sugars (e.g., table sugar, high fructose corn syrup, honey)

Most of the above are not part of the Paleolithic diet. That's the main reason the paleo diet helps control diabetes. Two items above, however, are paleo-approved: fruits and vegetables.

Many dietitians have been taught that you must eat at least 130 grams of carbohydrate daily to provide a rich, readily available source of energy—glucose, specifically—to your brain in particular, and other tissues. Millions of "low-carbers" (people with a low-carb way of eating) know that isn't right, having proven it to themselves by experience. I personally lived on 30 grams (or less) daily for four months without problems with my brain or other organs. (Well, my wife might argue about the brain issue.) I felt fine and had plenty of energy.

In healthy people, prediabetics, and mild diabetics not treated with medication, carbohydrate restriction rarely causes low blood sugar problems (hypoglycemia). But in other diabetics, carbohydrate restriction can lead to serious, even life-threatening, symptoms of hypoglycemia.

HYPOGLYCEMIA: RECOGNITION AND MANAGEMENT

Hypoglycemia is by far the most prominent risk for a diabetic on certain drugs starting a low-carb paleo diet. Hypoglycemia means an abnormally low blood sugar (under 60–70 mg/dl or 3.3–3.9 mmol/l) associated with symptoms such as weakness, malaise, anxiety, irritability, shaking, sweating, hunger, fast heart rate, blurry vision, difficulty concentrating, or dizziness. Symptoms often start suddenly and without obvious explanation. If not recognized and treated, hypoglycemia can lead to incoordination, altered mental status (fuzzy thinking, disorientation, confusion, odd behavior, lethargy), loss of consciousness, seizures, and even death (rare).

You can imagine the consequences if you develop fuzzy thinking or lose consciousness while driving a car, operating dangerous machinery, rock climbing, or scuba diving.

Your personal physician and other healthcare team members will teach you how to recognize and manage hypoglycemia. Immediate early stage treatment involves ingestion of glucose as the preferred treatment: 15 to 20 grams. You can get glucose tablets or paste at your local pharmacy without a prescription. Other carbohydrates will also work: six fl oz (180 ml) sweetened fruit juice, 12 fl oz (360 ml) milk, four tsp (20 ml) table sugar mixed in water, four fl oz (120 ml) soda pop, candy, etc. Fifteen to 30 grams of glucose or other carbohydrate should do the trick. Hypoglycemic symptoms respond within 20 minutes.

If level of consciousness is diminished such that the person cannot safely swallow, he will need a glucagon injection. Non-medical people can be trained to give the injection under the skin or into a muscle. Ask your doctor if you are at risk for severe hypoglycemia. If so, ask him for a prescription so you can get an emergency glucagon kit from a pharmacy.

Some people with diabetes, particularly after having the condition for many years, lose the ability to detect hypoglycemia just by the way they feel. This "hypoglycemia unawareness" is obviously more dangerous than being able to detect and treat hypoglycemia early on. Blood sugar levels may continue to fall and reach a life-threatening degree. Hypoglycemia unawareness can be caused by impairment of the nervous system (autonomic neuropathy) or by beta blocker drugs prescribed for high blood pressure or heart disease. People with hypoglycemia unawareness need to check blood sugars more frequently, particularly if driving a car or operating dangerous machinery.

Do not assume your sugar is low every time you feel a little hungry, weak, or anxious. Use your home glucose monitor for confirmation when able.

If you do experience hypoglycemia, discuss management options with your doctor: downward medication adjustment, shifting meal quantities or times, adjustment of exercise routine, eating more carbohydrates, etc. If you're trying to lose weight or control high blood sugars, reducing certain diabetic drugs makes more sense than eating more carbs. Eating at regular intervals three or four times daily may help prevent hypoglycemia. Spreading carbohydrate consumption evenly throughout the day may help. Someone most active during daylight hours as opposed to nighttime will generally do better eating carbs at breakfast and lunch rather than concentrating them at bedtime.

Your car is designed to run on gasoline. When you put diesel fuel into its tank, the results are disastrous for the engine. The same principle is true for us: We are designed to run best on the wild plant and animal foods that all humans gathered and hunted just 500 generations ago. The staples of today's diet—cereals, dairy product, refined sugars, fatty meats, and salted processed foods—are like diesel fuel to our body's metabolic machinery. These foods clog our engines, make us fat, and cause disease and ill health.

—Loren Cordain in *The Paleo Diet* (2001)

8
Diabetes Drug Dose Adjustments

Hypoglycemia is a major risk for diabetics taking certain diabetic drugs while on a carbohydrate-restricted diet. Serious, even life-threatening, symptoms of hypoglycemia may arise. This is dangerous territory.

Many classes of drugs used to treat diabetes have no risk of causing hypoglycemia. You've got to know what class of drug you're taking. The next chapter–Drugs for Diabetes–should help in that respect. If you have any doubt about whether your diabetic drug has the potential to cause hypoglycemia, ask your physician, pharmacist, or certified diabetes educator.

Remember, drugs have both generic and brand names. The names vary from country to country, as well as by manufacturer. Even the names of drug classes can be confusing. For instance, meglitinide drugs are sometimes just called glinides.

DRUGS THAT RARELY, IF EVER, CAUSE HYPOGLYCEMIA

Diabetics not being treated with pills or insulin rarely need to worry about hypoglycemia. That's usually true also for prediabetics. Yes, some type 2 diabetics control their condition with diet and exercise alone, without drugs.

Similarly, diabetics treated only with diet, metformin, colesevalam, sodium-glucose co-transport 2 inhibitor (SGLT2 inhibitor), and/or an alpha-glucosidase inhibitor (acarbose, miglitol) should not have much, if any, trouble with hypoglycemia. The DPP4-inhibitors (sitagliptan and saxagliptin) do not seem to cause low glucose levels, whether used alone or combined with metformin or a thiazoladinedione. Thiazolidinediones by themselves cause hypoglycemia in only 1 to 3% of users, but might cause a higher percentage in people on a reduced calorie diet. Bromocriptine may slightly increase the risk of hypoglycemia. GLP-1 analogues rarely cause hypoglycemia, but they can.

DRUGS THAT CAUSE HYPOGLYCEMIA

Regardless of diet, diabetics are at risk for hypoglycemia if they use any of the following drug classes. Also listed are a few of the individual drugs in some classes:
- insulins

- sulfonylureas: glipizide, glyburide, glimiperide, chlorpropamide, acetohexamide, tolbutamide
- meglitinides: repaglinide, nateglinide
- pramlintide plus insulin
- possibly GLP-1 analogues
- GLP-1 analogues (exanatide, liragultide, albiglutide, dulaglutide) when used with insulin, sufonylureas, or meglitinides
- possibly thiazolidinediones: pioglitazone, rosiglitazone
- possibly bromocriptine

DRUG ADJUSTMENTS TO AVOID HYPOGLYCEMIA

Diabetics considering or following a carbohydrate-restricted diet must work closely with their personal physician, dietitian, or certified diabetes educator to avoid hypoglycemia caused by the aforementioned classes of diabetic drugs.

Clinical experience with thousands of patients has led to generally accepted guidelines that help avoid hypoglycemia in diabetics on medications. A typical adult diabetic eating a standard "diabetic diet" is eating 225 to 300 grams of carbohydrate daily. Any significant reduction from that level could lead to hypoglycemia. The Paleobetic Diet will cut your carbs to the range of 40 to 80 grams of digestible carbohydrate. Common strategies for diabetics on hypoglycemia-inducing drugs and starting a low-carb diet include:
- reduce the insulin dose by a quarter or half
- change short-acting insulin to long-acting (such as glargine)
- stop the sulfonylurea, or reduce dose by a quarter or half

- reduce the thiazolidinedione by up to a half
- stop the meglitinide, or reduce the dose by up to a half
- if taking a GLP-1 analogue as the sole diabetes drug, either hold steady on the dose (particularly if blood sugars are running higher than optimal) or reduce dose by half
- monitor blood sugars frequently, at least until a stable pattern is established
- spread carbohydrate consumption evenly throughout the day

Management also includes frequent monitoring of glucose levels with a home glucose monitor, often four to six times daily. Common measurement times are before meals and at bedtime. It may be helpful to occasionally wake at 3 AM and check a sugar level. To see the effect of a particular food or meal on glucose level, check it one or two hours after eating. Keep a record. When eating patterns are stable, and blood sugar levels are reasonable and stable, monitoring can be done less often. When food consumption or exercise habits change significantly, check sugar levels more often.

If you're thinking that many diabetics on low-carb diets use fewer diabetic medications, you're right! That's probably a good thing since the long-term side effects of many of the drugs we use are unknown. Remember Rezulin (troglitazone)? Introduced in 1997, it was pulled off the U.S. market in 2001 because of fatal liver toxicity. In 2010, rosiglitazone was heavily restricted in the U.S. out of concern for heart toxicity.

I recommend you become the expert on the diabetic drugs you take. Don't depend solely on your physician. Do research at reliable sources and keep written notes. With a little effort, you could quickly surpass your doctor's knowledge of your specific drugs. What are the side effects? How common are they? How soon do they work? Any interactions with other drugs? What's the right dose, and how often can it be changed? Do you need blood tests to monitor for toxicity? How often? Who absolutely should not take this drug? Along with everything else your doctor has to keep up with, he prescribes about a hundred drugs on a regular basis. You only have to learn about two or three. It could save your life.

The deviation of man from the state in which he was originally placed by nature seems to have proved to him a prolific source of diseases.

—Edward Jenner (1749–1823), of smallpox vaccination fame

9
Drugs for Diabetes

We've never had so many pharmaceutical options for treating diabetes—12 different classes as of 2015. Most classes have more than one drug.

Diabetes medications are the major cause of hypoglycemia in people with diabetes. Blood sugars can drop dangerously low in people taking certain medications while cutting back on calorie consumption or reducing the amount of carbohydrates they eat. The more severe the carb or calorie restriction, the greater the risk of hypoglycemia.

WARNING!

THIS CHAPTER WILL PUT SUSCEPTIBLE
INDIVIDUALS TO SLEEP. DO NOT OPERATE
DANGEROUS MACHINERY OR DRIVE WHILE
READING.

If you don't take any drugs to control diabetes or prediabetes, you're free to skip this chapter. Otherwise, find your drugs herein and pay careful attention to those. Reading about the other drugs is likely to bore you; skip them. Note especially if your drugs are the ones that can cause low blood sugar. If so, you and your doctor may well have to reduce the medication dose—or even stop the drug—when you start the carbohydrate-restricted Paleobetic diet. The previous chapter has some tips on reducing drug dosages. As mentioned there, you need to become the expert on the diabetes drugs you take.

If you don't know your diabetes drug's name(s), go check the bottle now. Your pharmacist, personal physician, and diabetes nurse educator are indispensible if any doubts remain about your drug's name, class, or potential to cause hypoglycemia.

Be aware that drugs have both generic and brand names. For instance, metformin (a generic name) is sold under the brand name of Glucophage, among other brand names depending on the manufacturer or distributor. Complicating matters further is that generic and brand names vary from one country to the next. I practice medicine in the U.S., so U.S. names are the ones I'll use. I will always capitalize a brand name drug, but start generic names with lower case letters unless it's the first word of a sentence.

The U.S. Food and Drug Administration is charged with approving drugs as safe and effective, and monitoring ongoing safety once a drug is on the market. Doctors commonly prescribe drugs for purposes not approved by the FDA. That's called "off-label." However, for our purposes here, I've restricted my comments to FDA-approved uses.

You may be surprised to learn that the FDA's definition of a drug's "effectiveness" is simply whether it lowers hemoglobin A1c or blood sugar levels to a significant degree. In an ideal world, we would also judge effectiveness based on prolongation of life, improvement in quality of life, and prevention of diabetes complications such as kidney failure, amputations, blindness, nerve damage, heart attacks, and strokes. Unfortunately, we don't have proof for most of our drugs that they do any of that. Probably some of our drugs have harmful long-term effects that we don't even know about yet. Keep your eyes open.

Because we don't know how most of our diabetes drugs affect long-term health outcomes, I recommend my patients use lifestyle measures—mostly diet modification and exercise—to control their blood sugars as much as possible. We have proof that carbohydrate restriction lowers blood sugar levels and hemoglobin A1c. We know that a well-designed carbohydrate-restricted diet is compatible with a long, healthy life. We know that exercise is linked to improved long-term health outcomes. My strong opinion is that you're better off if you can control your blood sugars without resorting to drugs with unknown long-term effects. That being said, if you need drugs, use them.

Also, you should assume that nothing in this chapter applies to children, adolescents, pregnant women, and nursing mothers.

I strive to be as accurate as possible in sharing drug information with you, but I cannot guarantee accuracy. Anything I write today could be outdated tomorrow. Talk to your personal physician, pharmacist, or other qualified professional for detailed, up-to-date drug information.

141

LIST OF DRUG CLASSES

DRUGS FOR TYPE 1 DIABETES

Insulins
Pramlintide: Symlin

DRUGS FOR TYPE 2 DIABETES

Metformin: Glucophage, others
Sulfonylureas: glipizide, glyburide, glimiperide, others
Thiazolidinediones: rosiglitazone (Avandia) pioglitazone (Actos)
Dipeptidyl-peptidase-4 Inhibitors: sitagliptin (Januvia), saxagliptin (Onglyza), linagliptin (Tradjenta), alogliptin (Nesina), and vildagliptin
GLP-1 Analogues: exenatide (Byetta, Bydureon), liraglutide (Victoza), albiglutide (Tanzeum)
Insulins
Alpha-glucosidase Inhibitors: acarbose (Precose), miglitol (Glyset)
Meglitinides: repaglinide (Prandin), nateglinide (Starlix)
Pramlintide: Symlin
Colesevelam: WelChol
Dopamine Receptor Agonist: bromocriptine (Cycloset)
SGLT2 Inhibitors: canagliflozin, dapagliflozin, empagliflozin

INJECTABLE DRUGS FOR DIABETES

Insulins
Pramlintide: Symlin
GLP-1 Analogues: exenatide (Byetta, Bydureon),
liraglutide (Victoza), albiglutide (Tanzeum)

ORAL DRUGS FOR DIABETES

Metformin: Glucophage, others
Sulfonylureas: glipizide, glyburide, glimiperide,
others
Thiazolidinediones: rosiglitazone (Avandia),
pioglitazone (Actos)
Dipeptidyl-peptidase-4 Inhibitors: sitagliptin
(Januvia), saxagliptin (Onglyza), linagliptin
(Tradjenta), alogliptin (Nesina), and
vildagliptin
Alpha-glucosidase Inhibitors: acarbose (Pre-
cose), miglitol (Glyset)
Meglitinides: repaglinide (Prandin), nateglinide
(Starlix)
Colesevelam: WelChol
Dopamine Receptor Agonist: bromocriptine
(Cycloset)
SGLT2 Inhibitors: canagliflozin, dapagliflozin,
empagliflozin

Now let's look at the specific drug classes.

ALPHA-GLUCOSIDASE INHIBITORS

These are oral drugs for type 2 diabetes. They mainly decrease after-meal glucose levels. Alpha-
glucosidase inhibitors (AGIs) available in the U.S.
are acarbose (Precose) and miglitol (Glyset).

How do they work?

143

Many of the carbohydrates we eat are just basic sugar molecules joined to each other by chemical bonds, creating disaccharides, oligosaccharides, and polysaccharides. This is as true for bread and potatoes as it is for table sugar. To digest and absorb them, we have to break them down into the basic sugar molecules (monosaccharides). AGIs inhibit this breakdown process inside our intestine, decreasing the expected rise in blood sugar after we eat carbohydrates composed of chains of basic sugar molecules. They delay glucose absorption. So AGIs mainly decrease after-meal glucose levels.

Uses

They work alone or in combination with other diabetic medications, especially if the diet contains over 50% of energy in the form of complex carbohydrates. They are FDA-approved only for use in type 2 diabetes, but they have also been used in type 1.

Dosing

The starting dose is the same for both: 25 mg by mouth three times daily with the first bite of each main meal.

Side Effects

Belly pain, intestinal gas, diarrhea. Slight risk of hypoglycemia when it's used alone; higher risk when used with insulin shots or insulin secretagogues like sulfonylureas. If hypoglycemia occurs, you have to eat glucose to counteract it, not your usual non-glucose items because you won't absorb them properly.

Don't use if you have liver cirrhosis (don't use acarbose; miglitol is OK), kidney impairment, or intestinal problems.

BROMOCRIPTINE

Cycloset (bromocriptine mesylate) is a fairly recent FDA-approved oral drug for treatment of type 2 diabetes. It's a completely new approach that increases dopamine activity in the brain. It's the only drug in a class called dopamine receptor agonists.

Bromocriptine has been in use for many years to treat other conditions, so we may not see any of the unforeseen consequences that have led to so many drugs being pulled from the market a few years after FDA approval.

How does it work?

How it lowers glucose levels is not entirely clear, but it may reset or alter glucose metabolism in tissues outside the brain. Bromocriptine is an ergot derivative that increases dopamine activity in the brain. It improves after-meal glucoses without an increase in blood insulin levels. This is appealing since high insulin levels are implicated as a contributor to some chronic diseases.

Uses

It's for adults with type 2 diabetes and can be used alone or with certain other diabetes drugs. The other drugs used in clinical trials were mostly metformin and sulfonylureas, with less experience using it with thiazolidinediones. We know little about using it with insulin. Bromocriptine is not for type 1 diabetics or diabetic ketoacidosis. It lowers hemoglobin A1c by 0.6 to 0.9% (absolute decrease).

Dosing

Start with 0.8 mg every morning and increase by an additional tablet (0.8 mg) weekly up to 4.8 mg or the maximal tolerated dose (1.6 to 4.8 mg). Take all of it in the morning.

Side Effects

In clinical studies, the most common cause for discontinuation of the drug was nausea. It can cause drowsiness, fainting, blood pressure drops with standing (causing lightheadedness, fainting, weakness, or sweating), fatigue, vomiting, and headaches. Hypoglycemia is not much of a problem, if any, when bromocriptine is used as the sole diabetic medication. In other words, bromocriptine by itself may slightly increase the risk of hypoglycemia.

Don't use it if you take neuroleptic drugs, are a nursing mother, have syncopal migraines (that make you faint), have hypersensitivity to ergot-related drugs, or have a severe psychotic disorder.

COLESEVELAM

Colesevelam is used primarily to reduce elevated levels of LDL cholesterol. Sold in the U.S. as Wel-Chol, it's also an oral drug for type 2 diabetes. It's the only diabetes drug in a class called bile acid sequestrants.

How does it work? Unclear.

Uses

Colesevelam is FDA-approved for treatment of type 2 diabetes in conjunction with insulin or diabetic pills.

Dosing

Three tablets twice daily with meals, or six tablets once daily with a meal.

Side Effects

Constipation in one of every 10 users.

Don't use if you have serum triglycerides over 500 mg/dl (5.65 mmol/l), or have gastroparesis, other gastrointestinal motility disorders, risk factors for bowel obstruction, or recent major gastrointestinal procedures.

DIPEPTIDYL-PEPTIDASE-4 INHIBITORS

The dipeptidyl-peptidase-4 inhibitors available in the U.S. are sitagliptin (sold as Januvia), saxagliptin (sold as Onglyza), linagliptin (Tradjenta) and alogliptin (Nesina). Vildagliptin is available in other countries. So we don't choke on our tongues, let's just call this class DPP-4 inhibitors. They are oral drugs for type 2 diabetes.

How do they work?

DPP-4 inhibitors decrease both fasting and after-meal blood sugar levels primarily by increasing insulin release from pancreas beta cells. How they do it is complicated.

First off, you need to know that two gastrointestinal hormones levels—glucagon-like peptide-1 (GLP-1) and gastric inhibitory polypeptide—increase in response to a meal. These hormones increase insulin secretion by pancreas beta cells, suppress glucagon secretion from pancreas alpha cells after meals, help suppress glucose production by the liver, and improve glucose uptake by tissues outside the liver. GLP-1 also slows emptying by the stomach and reduces food intake. All this tends to lower glucose levels after meals.

If we could make these gut hormones hang around longer, their glucose-lowering action would be enhanced. How can we make them hang around and work longer? Simply suppress the enzyme that degrades them: dipeptidyl-peptidase-4. That's what DPP-4 inhibitors do.

The small intestine hormone GLP-1 is a major player in normal carbohydrate metabolism. GLP-1 levels, by the way, are decreased in type 2 diabetes.

For the DPP-4 inhibitors, we have no data on long-term safety, mortality, or diabetic complications.

Uses

Sitagliptin is FDA-approved as initial drug therapy for the treatment of type 2 diabetes, and as a second agent in those who do not respond to a single agent, such as metformin, a sulfonylurea, or a thiazolidinedione. It can also be used as a third agent when dual therapy with a sulfonylurea and metformin doesn't provide adequate blood sugar control.

Saxagliptin, linagliptin, and alogliptin are FDA-approved as initial drug therapy for the treatment of type 2 diabetes (in adults) or as add-on drugs for those who do not respond to a single drug, such as metformin, a sulfonylurea, or a thiazolidinedione. In case you're wondering, you wouldn't use several of the DPP-4 inhibitors at the same time. In the summer of 2012, the FDA approved linagliptin as an add-on drug for type 2 diabetics already taking insulin. Linagliptin and alogliptin haven't been studied in nursing or pregnant women; I'm not sure about sitagliptin and saxagliptin in those settings. Alogliptin is approved for combined use with metformin, pioglitazone, insulin, and perhaps sulfonylureas.

Dosing

The DPP-4 inhibitors are given by mouth. The usual dose of sitagliptin is 100 mg once daily, with reduction to 50 mg for moderate to severe kidney impairment and 25 mg for severe kidney impairment. The usual dose of saxagliptin is 2.5 or 5 mg once daily, with the 2.5 mg dose recommended for patients with moderate to severe kidney impairment. Linagliptin's dose is 5 mg daily, regardless of liver or kidney function. The alogliptin dose is 25 mg daily, with lower doses for those with kidney impairment.

Side Effects

Generally well-tolerated. No risk of hypoglycemia when used as the sole diabetes drug. They do not cause weight gain. Sitagliptin, linagliptin, and alogliptin might cause pancreatitis. Alogliptin may cause liver disease or abnormal liver function blood tests.

Don't use if you have moderate or severe kidney impairment (sitagliptin) or severe kidney impairment (saxagliptin).

Use sitagliptin or alogliptin with caution and careful monitoring if you have a history of pancreatitis.

GLP-1 ANALOGUES

These are injectable (subcutaneous) drugs for type 2 diabetes. GLP-1 analogues available in the U.S. are exenatide (sold as Byetta), liraglutide (Victoza), albiglutide (Tanzeum), and dulaglutide (Trulicity). They are sometimes referred to as GLP-1 receptor agonists. They are not considered first-choice drugs, but instead are typically used in combination with other drugs. Some can be used with insulin, others not.

Fun Fact for the diabetic version of Trivial Pursuit: Exenatide (Byetta) is a synthesized version of a protein initially discovered in the saliva of a lizard, the Gila monster.

How Do They Work?

It's complicated. First off, you need to know that a small intestine hormone, glucagon-like peptide-1 (GLP-1), is produced in response to a meal. This hormone increases insulin secretion by pancreas beta cells, suppresses glucagon after meals, inhibits emptying of the stomach, and inhibits appetite. Other effects are suppression of glucose production by the liver, and improved glucose uptake by tissues outside the liver. All this tends to lower blood sugar levels after meals.

The problem is that GLP-1 is quickly destroyed by an enzyme called DPP-4. We have available to us now chemicals similar to GLP-1, called GLP-1 analogues, that bind to the GLP-1 receptors and are resistant to degradation by the enzyme DPP-4. They essentially act like GLP-1, and they hang around longer.

GLP-1 levels, by the way, are decreased in type 2 diabetes.

The action of GLP-1 is dependent on blood sugar levels. If blood glucose is not elevated, GLP-1 doesn't go to work. From a practical viewpoint, this means that GLP-1 analogues, when used as the sole diabetes drug, rarely cause hypoglycemia.

We know little about long-term outcomes with these drugs, such as diabetic complications, health-related quality of life, or mortality.

Uses

Exenatide is FDA-approved for adults with type 2 diabetes who are not adequately controlled with metformin, sulfonylurea, or a thiazolidinedione (or a combination of these agents). It can be used with insulin glargine (e.g., Lantus). So it's an add-on drug, not approved for use by itself. The manufacturer cannot recommend its use with meal-time rapid-acting insulin since that hasn't been formally studied. Exenatide is a twice daily subcutaneous injection.

Once-weekly exenatide (Bydureon) was FDA-approved in January, 2012. It's not a first-line therapy. Don't use along with Byetta. In clinical trials it has been used along with metformin, sulfonylureas, and thiazolidinediones; by implication it seems to be OK to use Bydureon with those drugs. Use with insulin has not been studied and is not recommended by the manufacturer.

Liraglutide is FDA-approved for treatment of type 2 diabetes but is not recommended as initial therapy, although it does seem to be approved for use by itself. It has been used alone and also in combination with metformin, sulfonylurea, and/or thiazolidinediones. It's not approved for use with insulin therapy.

Albiglutide is for adult type 2 diabetes and can be used alone or with other drugs, but it's not a first-line agent. It was FDA-approved in 2014. It's a once weekly subcutaneous injection that can be used alone or in combination with metformin, glimiperide (and presumably other sulfonylureas), pioglitazone (and presumably other thiazoladinediones), and insulin.

Dulaglutide was FDA-approved for treatment of adults with type 2 diabetes in September, 2014. The once-weekly injection can be used by itself or in combination with metformin, glimiperide (and presumably other sulfonylureas), pioglitazone, and insulin lispro (e.g., Humalog, a rapid-acting insulin). It has not been tried with basal (long-acting) insulin. It's not a first-line drug.

Dosing

They are available only as subcutaneous injections (under the skin). Exenatide is twice daily, starting at 5 mcg within 60 minutes prior to a meal. After four weeks, the dose is increased to 10 mcg twice daily.

Bydureon is the U.S. trade name for a long-acting form of exenatide. The dose is 2 mg injected subcutaneously every seven days.

Liraglutide is a once daily subcutaneous injection starting at 0.6 mg, increasing to 1.2 mg after one week. It is given without regard to meals. Maximum dose is 1.8 mg/day.

Albiglutide is started at 30 mg subcutaneously, increasing to 50 mg if needed.

Dulaglutide starts at 0.75 mg and can be increased to 1.5 mg weekly.

Side Effects

GLP-1 analogues tend to cause nausea, vomiting, and diarrhea in as many as four in 10 users. The nausea typically improves over time. They tend to cause weight loss. They might cause pancreatitis, which is potentially life-threatening.

Hypoglycemia is rare unless they are used with insulin or an insulin secretagogue (a sulfonylurea or meglitinide).

Liraglutide and dulaglutide might cause thyroid cancer or tumors.

Dulaglutide may also cause abdominal pain, loss of appetite, dyspepsia, and fatigue.

Don't use if you have severe kidney impairment (exenatide), Multiple Endocrine Neoplasia syndrome (liraglutide), Multiple Endocrine Neoplasia syndrome type 2 (albiglutide and dulaglutide), or family history of medullary thyroid cancer (liraglutide, albiglutide, dulaglutide), or personal history of medullary thyroid cancer (albiglutide and dulaglutide).

Use GLP-1 analogues with caution if you have a history of pancreatitis or gastroparesis. Avoid dulaglutide in cases of severe pre-existing gastrointestinal disease.

Use liraglutide with caution in patients with kidney or liver impairment. Dulaglutide may be risky in patients with liver impairment.

None of these drugs have been tested in pregnant or nursing mothers; avoid use in those settings.

INSULINS

Insulin is life-saving for type 1 diabetics. Many type 2 diabetics will eventually, if not at the outset, need to take insulin for adequate control of blood sugars, which should help prevent diabetes complications.

How does it work?

Insulin is made by the healthy pancreas to keep blood sugars from rising above a fairly strict range: 70–140 mg/dl or 3.89–7.78 mmol/l. (It has many other actions as discussed elsewhere.) When we eat a meal containing carbohydrates (and proteins to a lesser extent), blood sugar starts to rise as we digest the carbs. Insulin drives the sugar into our body's cells for use as immediate energy or conversion to fat or glycogen as stored energy. About half of the daily insulin produced by a healthy body is "basal," meaning it's secreted into the bloodstream in a steady, low-volume amount, to keep the liver from making too much blood sugar (glucose), and for controlling fasting sugar levels. The other half is secreted in to the bloodstream in response to meals.

In type 2 diabetes, the body's tissues, at first, are resistant to the effect of insulin. So the pancreas has to secrete more than usual to get the job done, a condition called hyperinsulinemia. As the illness progresses, the pancreas cannot keep up with demand for more insulin and starts to "burn out," producing less insulin. As the burn out process continues, many diabetics need to start insulin injections. (These are generalities; there are exceptions.)

Type 1 diabetics have an immune-mediated process that destroys the insulin-producing beta cells in the pancreas. Once the disease is well-established, the pancreas secretes no insulin at all. Type 1 diabetics will die without injected insulin, although the process could take weeks, months, or even a few years.

We could break down the various insulins into two types: human (identical in structure to human insulin) and analogs (minor molecular modifications to the usual human insulin molecule). The two human insulins are NPH and "regular." All the others are analogs. But most people don't care about that.

It's more helpful to distinguish insulins by the timing of their action:
- Rapid acting: lispro (e.g., Lantus), aspart (e.g., Novolog), glulisine (e.g., Apidra), inhaled insulin (e.g., Afrezza)
- Short acting: regular (e.g., Novolin R, Humulin R)
- Intermediate to long acting: NPH, glargine (e.g., Lantus), determir (e.g., Levemir), NPL (neutral protamine lispro)

Rapid-acting insulins have an onset of action between five and 15 minutes, peak effect in 30 to 90 minutes, and duration of action of two to four hours.

155

Short-acting "regular insulin" has onset in 30 minutes, peaks in two to four hours, and works for five to eight hours.

Intermediate to long-acting insulins start working in two hours, don't have a well-defined peak of action, and keep working for 20 or more hours (glargine) or for six to 23 hours (detemir).

All these times are gross approximations. Once the insulin is injected into the fat below the skin, it has to be absorbed into the bloodstream and transported to the tissues where it does its magic. Lots of factors affect this process. For instance, the thicker the fat tissue at the injection site, the slower the absorption. Absorption tends to be faster from the abdominal wall, slower from the arms, even slower from the thighs or buttocks. Absorption can vary from day to day in an individual even when injection site and technique are identical.

As you might have guessed, the short- and rapid-acting insulins are usually injected before a meal in anticipation of blood sugar rising as food is digested. The intermediate- and long-acting insulins imitate the healthy body's "basal" insulin.

Manufacturers also supply premixed insulins, combining intermediate or long-acting insulin with a short- or rapid-acting insulin. Examples are Humalog 75/25, Humulin 70/30, and Novolog 70/30.

In case you're wondering, modern insulin injections are barely painful, if at all.

In 2014, the U.S. Food and Drug Administration approved use of an inhaled rapid-acting insulin called Afrezza. As of the time of publication of this book, very few U.S. patients and doctors have experience with it. Afrezza is for adults with either type 1 or 2 diabetes. It should not be used in smokers or those with chronic lung disease such as asthma or chronic obstructive lung disease (COPD). The most common side effects are hypoglycemia, cough, and throat pain. Type 1 diabetics still need to take a basal (long-acting) insulin injections once or twice daily. As far as I can tell, the type 2 diabetics in the pre-approval clinical studies were all taking one or more oral diabetic drugs in addition to the Afrezza; the inhaled insulin was an add-on drug. The manufacturer recommends a test of lung function before starting the drug, to identify folks with lung disease who shouldn't inhale insulin. The test is called spirometry or FEV-1 (forced expiratory volume in 1 second). Moreover, spirometry should be repeated six months after start of the drug, then yearly thereafter.

Another form of inhaled insulin—Exubera—was on the U.S. market in 2006 and discontinued by the manufacturer the next year. The problem may have been poor sales or a concern about lung cancer.

Dose and Selection of Insulin

Anyone taking insulin must work closely with a physician or diabetes nurse educator on proper dosing, injection technique, and recognition and management of hypoglycemia (low blood sugar). Many type 2 diabetics get started just with an intermediate or long-acting insulin once or twice daily, with or without diabetes drugs by mouth. If and when the illness progresses, rapid-acting insulin may be added later. A typical insulin regimen for a type 1 diabetic would be one or two daily injections of a long-acting insulin, plus three or four rapid-acting insulin injections around meals and snack time.

Another less common insulin regimen involves a battery-operated pump worn continuously, which infuses basal amounts of insulin plus mealtime boluses.

From a practical viewpoint, by far the most common and worrisome side effect of insulin is hypoglycemia.

MEGLITINIDES

Meglitinides, also called glinides, are oral drugs for type 2 diabetes. Two are available in the U.S.: repaglinide is sold as Prandin, and nateglinide as Starlix. They have about the same effectiveness as sulfonylureas, but are considerably more expensive. Glinides work mostly to reduce sugar levels after meals.

We don't know if these drugs affect longevity or long-term diabetes complication rates. The same can be said about most diabetes drugs.

How do they work?

Meglitinides increase the output of insulin by the pancreas beta cells into the bloodstream. In that respect they are similar to sulfonylurea drugs, so the two classes are sometimes lumped together as insulin secretagogues. If the pancreas produces no insulin at all—as in nearly all cases of type 1 diabetes—these drugs won't work.

Repaglinide and nateglinide increase insulin secretion by the pancreas, working faster than sulfonylureas. They don't last as long as sulfonylureas, which may help avoid hypoglycemia.

Uses

They may be used alone or in combination with certain other diabetic drugs. Since they have the same mechanism of action, sulfonylureas and meglitinides would not normally be used together. In combination therapy, you want to use drug classes that work by different mechanisms.

Dosing

Starting dose for repaglinide is 0.5 mg by mouth before each meal. Maximum dose is 4 mg before each meal.

Nateglinide: 120 mg by mouth immediately before each meal.

Side Effects

Hypoglycemia is the most common and potentially serious adverse effect of the meglitinides, but may be less common than with sulfonylureas. Weight gain is common.

Precautions...

Nateglinide: Use with great caution, if at all, in the setting of severe kidney disease and moderate to severe liver disease.

Repaglinide: Use cautiously in severe kidney and liver disease.

METFORMIN

Metformin is a major drug for treatment of type 2 diabetes. In fact, it's usually the first choice when a drug is needed. It is the only drug in its class (bi-quanides).

How does it work?

In short, metformin decreases glucose output by the liver. The liver produces glucose (sugar) either by breaking down glycogen stored there or by manu-facturing glucose from smaller molecules and at-oms. The liver then kicks the glucose into the bloodstream for use by other tissues. Insulin inhib-its this function of the liver, thereby keeping blood sugar levels from getting too high. Metformin im-proves the effectiveness of insulin in suppressing sugar production. In other words, it works primarily by decreasing the liver's production of glucose.

Physicians talk about metformin as an "insulin sen-sitizer," primarily in the liver but also to a lesser ex-tent in peripheral tissues such as fat tissue and muscle. It doesn't work without insulin in the body.

Metformin typically lowers fasting blood sugar by about 20% and hemoglobin A1c by 1.5% (absolute decrease, not relative).

When used as the sole diabetic medication, metfor-min is associated with decreased risk of death and heart attack, compared to therapy with sulfonylure-as, thiazolidinediones, alpha-glucosidase inhibitors, and meglitinides.

Metformin tends to cause a bit of weight loss and improved cholesterol levels. Insulin and sulfonylu-rea therapy, on the other hand, typically lead to weight gain of 8–10 pounds (4 kg) on aver-age.

Uses

Metformin works by itself, but can also be used in combination with most of the other diabetic medications. It's usually taken once or twice daily.

Dose

Starting dose is typically 500 mg taken with the evening meal. The dose can be increased every week or two. If more than 500 mg/day is needed, the second dose—500 mg—is usually given with breakfast. The usual effective maximum dose is 2,000 mg daily.

Side Effects

Metallic taste, diarrhea, belly pain, loss of appetite. Possible impaired absorption of vitamin B12, leading to anemia. When used alone, it has very little risk of hypoglycemia. Rare: lactic acidosis.

Don't use metformin if you have impaired kidney function, congestive heart failure of a degree that requires drug therapy (this is debatable), active liver disease, or chronic alcohol abuse.

PRAMLINTIDE

Pramlintide is an injectable drug sold in the U.S. as Symlin. It's only used in patients already taking meal-time rapid-acting insulin. It's particularly useful in preventing large increases in blood sugar in the several hours after a meal. Pramlintide may have a role in treatment of overweight type 2 diabetics inadequately controlled on insulin, or who experience weight gain refractory to diet and exercise. Type 1s can use it, too.

Class: amylin analogue.

How does it work?

Amylin is a hormone stored in pancreas beta cells and is secreted along with insulin. It affects glucose levels by several mechanisms, including slowed stomach emptying, regulation of glucagon secretion after meals, and by reducing food intake. Amylin and insulin levels rise and fall together in a healthy body, working jointly to control blood sugar levels. Amylin is relatively deficient in many cases of type 2 diabetes.

Pramlintide is a chemical similar in structure to amylin and causes similar effects. It allows insulin therapy to more easily match the body's needs in the after-meal period. It also promotes modest weight loss in obese patients.

Pramlintide therapy reduces hemoglobin A1c by 0.5 to 1% (absolute decrease, not relative).

We have no data on long-term health outcomes with this drug.

Uses

Pramlintide is FDA-approved for use in both type 1 diabetes and insulin-requiring type 2 diabetes. It can be used with metformin and/or sulfonylureas as long as insulin is also part of the regimen. It's probably best not to use it with exenatide and other GLP-1-based therapies.

Dosing

It's injected subcutaneously just before meals, starting with 60 mcg in type 2 diabetics. To avoid hypoglycemia at the start of treatment, the pre-meal rapid-acting or mixed-acting insulin dose is usually reduced by half. Pramlintide should only be administered before meals that contain at least 30 grams of carbohydrate or 250 calories. The maximum dose is 120 mcg with each meal.

For type 1 diabetics, the initial dose is 15 mcg subcutaneously immediately prior to meals. The dose can be increased every three days in 15 mcg increments up to a target dose of 30–60 mcg. Again, to avoid hypoglycemia, the dose of rapid-acting and mixed-acting insulin preparations should be reduced by half.

Side Effects

Nausea is the most common side effect but clears up in a few weeks. Pramlintide by itself does not cause hypoglycemia, but since it is always used with injectable insulin, hypoglycemia may occur—usually within three hours.

Don't use if you have gastroparesis or hypoglycemia unawareness.

SULFONYLUREAS

Sulfonylureas (SUs) in 2015 are still the most widely used drugs for treatment of type 2 diabetes. They are not for type 1s. At least six different SUs are in common usage in the U.S., including glipizide, glimiperide, and glyburide. They are often prescribed for patients who do not respond adequately to lifestyle modification and are intolerant of metformin, the usual first-choice drug.

Sulfonlylureas make the pancreas beta cells secrete more insulin into the bloodstream. The other drugs that do this are the meglitinides; these two classes are sometimes lumped together as insulin secretagogues. The sulfonylureas are less expensive than meglitinides.

Metiglinides (repaglinide and nateglinide) have about the same effectiveness as SUs, but they work faster. They don't last as long as sulfonylureas, which may help avoid hypoglycemia. These two "glinides" work mostly to reduce sugar levels after meals.

We don't know if SUs affect death rates.

How do they work?

Sulfonylureas increase the pancreas's production of insulin after a meal (second phase insulin secretion). If the pancreas beta cells are no longer producing any insulin, SUs won't work. SUs decrease fasting blood sugar by about 20% and hemoglobin A1c by 1 or 2% (absolute, not relative).

Uses

Sulfonylureas may be used alone or in combination with certain other diabetic drugs. Since they have the same mechanism of action, sulfonylureas and meglitinides would not normally be used together. In combination therapy, you want to use drug classes that work by different mechanisms.

Dosing

SU dose depends on the particular one used. Some are taken by mouth once daily, others twice.

Side Effects

Hypoglycemia is the most severe adverse effect of the sulfonylureas. The duration of hypoglycemia seen with SUs is often much longer than you would predict by how much drug is in the bloodstream. Hypoglycemia is more common with the longer-acting drugs, such as glyburide and chlorpropamide. There is some concern that sulfonylureas are linked to poorer outcomes after a heart attack. SUs occasionally cause nausea, skin reactions, and elevations of liver function tests. Weight gain is common.

When used with insulin or thiazolidinediones, these sulfonylurea adverse effects are more likely to appear: weight gain, fluid retention, and congestive heart failure.

Precautions: Consult your personal physician or pharmacist.

THIAZOLIDINEDIONES

Thiazolidinediones are more easily referred to as TZDs or glitazones. Compared to the usual first-choice drug for type 2 diabetes (metformin), the TZDs are significantly more expensive. They are not type 1 drugs.

Remember that drug names—both generic and brand—may vary depending on country and manufacturer. In the U.S., rosiglitazone is sold as Avandia; pioglitazone as Actos.

165

How do they work?

In short, TZDs increase glucose utilization and decrease glucose production, leading to lower blood sugar levels. They sensitize several tissues to the effect of insulin. Insulin, among other actions, helps put circulating blood sugar into our muscles, fat cells, and (to a lesser extent) liver cells. So blood sugar levels fall. Thiazolidinediones make these tissues more sensitive to this effect of insulin. Insulin also suppresses glucose production by the liver, an effect enhanced by TZDs. They reduce insulin resistance.

TZDs may also help preserve pancreas beta cell function. Beta cells produce insulin.

They reduce both fasting and after-meal glucose levels. Fasting blood sugar drops and average of 40 mg/dl. Hemoglobin A1c falls by 1 to 1.5% (absolute, not relative).

TZDs tend to improve blood lipids: lower triglycerides, higher HDL cholesterol, decreased small, dense LDL cholesterol. Pioglitazone has the more pronounced effect.

On a cellular level, they activate peroxisome proliferator-activated receptor-gamma, so they are sometimes referred to as PPAR-gamma agonists. Pioglitazone also affects PPAR-alpha.

Uses

TZDs can be used alone or in combination with insulin, metformin, and sulfonylureas in people with type 2 diabetes.

Dosing

Note that onset of action is delayed by several weeks, perhaps as many as 8–12 weeks.

Pioglitazone: Start at 15–30 mg/day by mouth. Maximum dose is 45 mg/day.

Rosiglitizone: Start at 4 mg/day by mouth. After 8–12 weeks, dose may be increased to 8 mg/day.

Side Effects

Weight gain is fairly common, through both fluid retention and increase in fat tissue. Weight gain with pioglitazone, for example, is around 6–12 pounds (3–5 kg). Mild anemia and puffy feet and hands (edema from fluid retention) are also seen. Fluid retention may ultimately cause congestive heart failure. This drug-induced fluid retention does not respond very well to fluid pills (diuretics).

The combination of insulin injections and TZD may increase the risk of heart failure.

Some studies suggest that rosiglitazone increases the risk of heart attacks, heart failure, and premature death. That's why the Food and Drug Administration in 2011 drastically curtailed use of the drug. The FDA re-examined the data in 2013 and decided that rosiglitazone didn't increase cardiovascular risk after all. Nevertheless, many physicians still prefer rosiglitazone's competitor, pioglitazone (Actos).

Preliminary data suggest a link between bladder cancer and pioglitazone.

TZDs are associated with increased risk for broken bones, perhaps doubling the risk.

Macular edema—manifested by blurry vision—may occur infrequently.

When used as the sole diabetic medication, TZDs do not cause hypoglycemia. But when used with insulin injections or insulin secretagogues, low blood sugar can occur.

Don't use if you have a significant degree of congestive heart failure or active liver disease. Even a history of heart failure may be a reason to avoid TZDs. TZDs should probably not be used in women with low bone density or anyone else prone to fractures.

SGLT2 INHIBITORS

SGLT2 stands for sodium-glucose co-transport 2. These are oral drugs for type 2 diabetes in adults. In March, 2013, the U.S. Food and Drug Administration approved the first agent in the newest class of diabetes drugs: canagliflozin. It's sold in the U.S. as Invokana. In January 2014 the second drug in this class was approved: dapagliflozin or Farxiga. Finally, empagliflozin (Jardiance) was approved for sale in August, 2014. More SGLT2 inhibitors are in the pipeline.

How Do They Work?

Our kidneys filter glucose (sugar) out of our bloodstream, then reabsorb that glucose back into the bloodstream. (Don't ask me why.) SGLT2 inhibitors impair that reabsorption process, allowing some glucose to be excreted in our urine. You could call it a diuretic effect. Dapagliflozin at a dose of 10 mg/day, for example, causes the urinary loss of 70 grams of glucose daily.

Uses

These drugs are for adults with type 2 diabetes, to be used in combination with diet and exercise. They can be used alone or in combination with insulin, metformin, sulfonylureas, or pioglitazone. Dapagliflozin has also been tested in combination with sitagliptin, a DPP4-inhibitor. Clinical experience in combination with other diabetes drugs is very limited.

Dose

Canagliflozin starts at 100 mg by mouth daily, taken before the first meal of the day. Dose can be increased to 300 mg daily. Dapagliflozin dosing starts at 5 mg by mouth every morning, with or without food, and can be increased up to 10 mg once daily. Empagliflozin starts at 10 mg every morning, increasing to 25 every AM if needed.

Side Effects

The most common side effects are vaginal yeast infections (about 5% of women), urinary tract infections, and penile yeast infections (e.g., balanitis). Also noted are increased urination, and dizziness or fainting from low blood pressure after arising to stand (orthostatic hypotension). The low blood pressures are related to a diuretic effect (increased urination) of this class.

Hypoglycemia (low blood sugar) is quite uncommon, perhaps nonexistent, unless these drugs are used with other drugs that often cause hypoglycemia, such as insulin and insulin secretagogues (like sulfonylureas and meglitinides).

High potassium levels have been seen with canagliflozin. All three drugs may cause elevation of LDL cholesterol ("bad cholesterol").

Dapagliflozin and empagliflozin can cause elevations of creatinine in the blood, a warning that kidney function may be worsening.

Canagliflozin seems to promote weight loss and lower blood pressure, which may be welcomed by some.

Don't use if you...

- have diabetic ketoacidosis
- are pregnant or planning to get pregnant
- have advanced or severe kidney disease
- have severe kidney impairment (glomerular filtration rate under 60 ml/min/1.73 m-squared, at least for dapagliflozin)
- have type 1 diabetes
- are on dialysis
- are a nursing mother
- for dapagliflozin: active bladder cancer (and use caution if you have history of bladder cancer)

10
Daily Life With Paleo Eating

This chapter will give you an approach to overcoming the common problems linked to a carbohydrate-restricted paleo way of eating. The coping mechanisms here are not exhaustive, and at times you will need to figure out for yourself what works for you and your unique circumstances.

In order, here's what's ahead:

1. Learning to cook
2. More paleo diet recipes and cookbooks
3. Short-term physical effects
4. Shopping for food
5. Dining out
6. Cheating
7. Sweet cravings
8. Holidays
9. Hunger
10. Record-keeping
11. Weight-loss tips

1. LEARNING TO COOK

I don't boil eggs very often. When I do, I have to look up how to do it. Do you start with the eggs in cold water, or boil the water and then add the eggs? How long to boil? What's the trick to making them easy to peel? You can search the Internet for cooking instructions or acquire a basic time-tested cookbook to keep on hand. Here are a few:

- *Joy of Cooking: 75th Anniversary Edition* by Rombauer and Becker
- *How to Cook Everything: 2,000 Simple Recipes for Great Food* by Mark Bittman
- *The New Best Recipes* by Cook's Illustrated
- *Betty Crocker Cookbook: Everything You Need to Know to Cook Today.*

Unfortunately, I've noticed that lots of young 'uns were not taught how to cook when they were growing up. That's 'cause Mom or Dad picked up dinner at Burger King on the way home from work. Our culture of convenience has made it too easy for us to eat over-processed industrial food. I'm as guilty as the next guy. I think convenience foods are one reason so many of us are fat. If you're lucky, you may have a friend or relative willing to take you under their wing and teach you some basic cooking skills.

2. MORE PALEO DIET RECIPES AND COOKBOOKS

The last few years have seen an explosion of paleo diet cookbooks. Some of them assume you know how to boil water and what "braising" means. Others don't. Most of them, unfortunately, don't provide any nutritional analysis of the recipes. In other words, you won't know how many carbohydrates are in each serving, which is a major problem if you have diabetes. Some diabetics also find it helpful to know protein grams, fat grams, and calories. I'm aware of only three paleo diet cookbooks that provide adequate nutritional analysis for a diabetic:

- *500 Paleo Recipes* by Dana Carpender
- *Primal Blueprint Quick and Easy Meals* by Mark Sisson and Jennifer Meier
- *Practical Paleo* by Diane Sanfilippo (but you have to visit BalancedBites.com (48) for the nutritional analysis)

The Primal Blueprint book isn't "pure paleo" in that some of the recipes include dairy products like butter, cream, and full-fat yogurt. That's a minor quibble. The book has an oatmeal substitute I'm anxious to try: Primal Hot Cereal.

I've heard good things about several other paleo diet cookbooks. Evolutionary Psychiatrist Dr. Emily Deans and others praise *Well Fed* by Melissa Joulwan. There's also a *Well Fed 2* that I'm not familiar with. Check out *Everyday Paleo* and *Everyday Paleo Family Cookbook* by Sarah Fragoso. Loren Cordain brings us *The Real Paleo Diet Cookbook* (2015) and *The Paleo Diet Cookbook* (2010). If their blog is any indication, *Nom Nom Paleo* by Michelle Tam and Henry Fong should be wonderful. *The Primal Blueprint Cookbook* by Mark Sisson and Jennifer Meier has great reviews (again, it's paleo plus milk products). When you find a recipe you like, you can do your own nutritional analysis at websites like FitDay.com.

Most of the paleo cookbook authors have websites that share some free recipes so you can get an idea what's in the book before you pull the trigger.

WEBSITES WITH FREE PALEO-STYLE RECIPES

Unless noted, these don't provide nutritional analysis such as carb grams per serving.

- The Clothes Make the Girl (Melissa Joulwan) http://www.theclothesmakethegirl.com
- Whole Life Eating http://www.wholelifeeating.com
- Nom Nom Paleo (Michelle Tam) http://nomnompaleo.com
- Julianne's Paleo and Zone Nutrition (Julianne Taylor) http://paleozonenutrition.com
- The Paleo Diet (Loren Cordain et al) http://thepaleodiet.com
- Paleoista (Nell Stephenson) http://paleoista.com
- Everyday Paleo (Sarah Fragoso) http://everydaypaleo.com
- Catalyst Athletics http://catalystathletics.com (Bingo! *Includes basic nutrient analysis*)
- PaleoFood Recipe Collection http://www.paleofood.com
- Paleo Plan http://www.paleoplan.com
- Stalkerville http://stalkerville.net
- Perfect Health Diet (Paul and Shou-Ching Jaminet) http://perfecthealthdiet.com
- Diabetes Warrior (Steve Cooksey) http://diabetes-warrior.net
- Diane Sanfilippo http://balancedbites.com (*Includes nutritional analysis* for recipes in her cookbook, *Practical Paleo*)

DIY NUTRITIONAL ANALYSIS

Doing your own nutritional analysis, mostly for digestible carb grams, is a hassle. It doesn't take much intelligence, just time and attention to detail. That's why it's not usually done for non-diabetic recipes and cookbooks. Remember, most folks end up eating the same 10 or 12 meals over and over. That may sound boring and you think you're a special snowflake that surely eats more variety. But odds are, you don't have more variety. (Don't count the turkey you eat once a year as one of your regular meals.) Once you determine your desired dozen meals, it may well be worth your time to do the nutritional analysis. In fact, you may get by with calculating only the digestible carb grams per serving (also called net carbs). Then ensure you eat a good variety of protein foods, nuts, vegetables, and fruits following the Paleobetic Diet guidelines. The rest of the nutrients will probably fall into line. To do your own nutritional analysis, you can spend hundreds or thousands of dollars for dietitian-level software, or you can use free online resources such as:

- FitDay (http://www.fitday.com)
- SELFNutritionData
  (http://nutritiondata.self.com)
- USDA National Nutrient Database
  (http://ndb.nal.usda.gov)
- SparkRecipes
  (http://recipes.sparkpeople.com/recipe-calculator.asp)

You need to know the digestible or net carb grams per serving of any recipe you try. If not provided for you, you can do a full nutritional analysis of any recipe at FitDay, SELF-NutritionData, or SparkRecipes (see above). The SELFNutritionData database probably isn't updated regularly, which could be a problem. I use the USDA database for confirmation and clarification. I like FitDay quite a bit. It's set up to analyze a full days' worth of eating. To analyze your recipe there, just enter all the ingredients as if that's all you're eating for the day. It will make sense when you visit the site.

Don't forget that you may also have access to a dietitian who can design and analyze your 10 or 12 repetitive meals for you. Dietitians are invaluable resources. My favorite registered dietitian, Franziska Spritzler, does consultations by phone and online (e.g., via Skype) as well as in-person. For details, see:
http://www.lowcarbdietitian.com/nutrition-services.html

LOW-CARB RECIPES

The low-carb community is a great resource for carbohydrate-restricted dieters. Many low-carb recipes are paleo-compliant, while many are not. You'll find both in the same cookbook. Non-diabetic paleo dieters often eat fruits and starchy vegetables or tubers (e.g., potatoes) that low-carbers would eschew. Both groups avoid grains. Traditional low-carbers eat non-paleo items like hard cheese, butter, green beans and snow peas (legumes), and artificial sweeteners. Otherwise there's a fair amount of overlap between the two camps. Good news: The low-carbers almost always provide carb grams per serving. If you're pure paleo, just ignore the low-carb recipes that use milk products (cheese, butter, cream), legumes (green beans, snow peas), and artificial sweeteners. Check out these sources for recipes:

- *Low-Carbing Among Friends*, volumes 1 through 4 by Jennifer Eloff et al. (http://low-carb-news.blogspot.com)
- *500 Low-Carb Recipes, 200 Low-Carb Slow Cooker Recipes, 15-Minute Low-Carb Recipes,* and *1001 Low-Carb Recipes* by Dana Carpender (http://holdthetoast.com)
- DAR, a type 2 diabetic, shares her favorite low-carb recipes at http://dardreams.wordpress.com
- Chef Barrae has posted hundreds of low-carb recipes at her blog: Unrestricted Tastes on Restricted Diets: Distinctive Diabetic Recipes (htt://chefbarrae.blogspot.com)
- The message boards at Low Carb Friends (http://www.lowcarbfriends.com)
- Active Low-Carbers Forum (http://forum.lowcarber.org)
- Laura Dolson's About.com: Low Carb Diets blog (http://lowcarbdiets.about.com)

3. SHORT-TERM PHYSICAL EFFECTS

Low-carb paleo eating is quite safe in the vast majority of generally healthy people. However, you need to be aware of problems that may crop up.

Low Blood Sugar

This is by far the biggest risk for a diabetic switching from a typical diabetic diet to low-carb paleo eating. You'll be reducing your carbohydrate intake from 200–300 grams a day down to 45–80 grams. Since ingested carbohydrates are normally the main source of blood sugar, a marked cut in consumption tends to reduce blood sugar levels, even in people who don't have diabetes or prediabetes. Symptoms of low blood sugar (hypoglycemia) are rare in healthy people starting a low-carb diet. But hypoglycemia is much more common and potentially serious in diabetics taking certain medications. See chapter seven for a thorough review.

Malaise and Fatigue

These are not common but may occur early-on, and are temporary. You're switching from a carbohydrate-based energy metabolism to fat-based. This body re-boot may cause a sense of mild malaise, easy fatigue, low energy, achiness, and dizziness. Some folks have the entire syndrome, others just parts. It starts on the second or third day of the diet and may last for several days, a week at the most. People with diabetes need to make sure the symptoms are not caused by low blood sugar by using their home glucose monitor.

Regarding low energy and easy fatigue, people who are used to exercising or working vigorously may notice that they can't perform at their prior workload, an effect that may be noticeable for two to four weeks. They may need to cut back the intensity of their work-outs temporarily. The first few weeks of low-carb eating are not a good time to start a vigorous exercise program.

Malaise and fatigue are temporary. They're proof that your body is going through a watershed moment. Tough it out—you'll be glad you did.

Leg Cramps

These are rare but may occur in the first few weeks or months. They tend to happen at night, even waking people from sleep. While not serious, they can be painful. Cramps are often prevented by taking supplemental magnesium, potassium, calcium, or a combination. If they persist, see your doctor for a blood test of these minerals.

A stretching exercise may prevent leg cramps: 1) Stand about two or three feet away from a wall (measured at the toes) and keep your feet planted in one spot, 2) lean forward against the wall and use your outstretched arms and hands to keep your body from hitting the wall, 3) keeping your trunk and legs in a straight line, bend your elbows to let your head approach the wall, 4) notice the slight tensing and stretching of the calf muscles (this may be slightly uncomfortable but shouldn't be painful), 5) hold that position for 10 seconds, 6) then stand up straight and relax a while, 7) repeat steps 1 through 5 for five or ten times. For nocturnal leg cramps, do this stretching just before bedtime.

Low Blood Pressure

The Paleobetic Diet is relatively low in salt compared to the way most people eat. This could cause a lowering of blood pressure. Symptoms of excessively low blood pressure include dizziness, lightheadedness, weakness, fainting, and fatigue. You may notice these only when going from sitting to standing, or from lying to standing. If you take drugs to lower your blood pressure, the dosage may need to be reduced to prevent excessively low blood pressure.

If low blood pressure is causing the symptom, we usually find a systolic blood pressure under 90 mmHg. "Systolic pressure" is the top or first number in a blood pressure reading such as 125/85 (systolic pressure is 125). The only way to tell if the aforementioned symptoms are related to blood pressure is to check a blood pressure with an accurate monitor, which most of us don't have at home or work. Perhaps you could borrow a friend's. Alternatively, check your blood pressure at your doctor's office or one of the free machines in many pharmacies and supermarkets. In those settings, a systolic pressure under 100 mmHg, even if you feel fine, suggests that your pressure at other times is under 90. Low blood pressures often responds to an increase in salt and water consumption, such as half a teaspoon daily mixed in water or used on food.

Did you notice that low blood pressure symptoms overlap with low blood sugar symptoms? Sometimes the only way to tell the difference is to check your blood sugar level.

If you ever feel like you're about to faint, the best immediate actions is to lie down. If the impending faint is caused by low blood pressure, lying down will improve blood flow to your brain within seconds and may well prevent a loss of consciousness.

4. SHOPPING

Finding food for the Paleobetic diet shouldn't be a problem. Specific recommended foods are readily available at supermarkets. People committed long-term to the low-carb way of eating often get into baking or cooking with low-carb components that may be a bit harder to find. An example is almond flour, used as a substitute for wheat flour. You may find low-carb products at local stores or available on the Internet (e.g., Netrition.com).

You'll find a grocery shopping list for the Paleobetic diet at this URL:

https://paleodiabetic.files.wordpress.com/2014/04
/paleobetic-diet-shopping-list.pdf

How to choose a fresh fish for cooking:

1. Sniff it. Pass if it smells fishy, nasty, or pungent.
2. Check for clear, dark eyes. Pass if eyes are dull, gray, and sunken.
3. Does it look or feel slimy? Take a pass.
4. Skin should be moist and shiny, almost metallic.
5. Flesh should be firm, not mushy. Press it with your finger—it shouldn't leave an imprint.
6. Look for bright red gills.
7. Cook within a day or two.

Canned meats and fish are time-savers and often less expensive than fresh, raw products. Worried about mercury poisoning from fish? I've been practicing medicine for 30 years and haven't seen a case of it yet. Canned sardines are available with sauces such as tomato, jalapeno, or mustard—just be sure it doesn't add more than a couple carb grams per 4-ounce (113 g) serving. Also watch out for added carbs in canned meats. Man-made processed meats—sausages, Spam, bacon, liverwurst, or ham, for example—may have unacceptably high added carbs: if it's got over 2–3 g of carbs per 3 or 4-ounce (85–113 g) serving, take a pass and stick with natural meats.

Canned vegetables are usually OK, too. Consider canned asparagus and spinach, for example. These are often criticized for their salt content, but the Paleobetic Diet is naturally low in salt and tends to lower blood pressure, so you don't have to worry about the salt in canned vegetables. Frozen vegetables are also conveniently boiled-in-the-bag or microwaved. Also consider frozen fruits like strawberries.

Food manufacturers are finally responding to consumer requests for truly "natural" foods with less man-made ingredients such as high fructose corn syrup (HFCS; pure carbohydrate). Search the shelves of your supermarket and you'll find ketchup and picante sauce with all-natural ingredients and no HFCS.

Keep your refrigerator and cupboards stocked with the foods you'll be eating, particularly if others in your household are eating regular foods that will tempt you to return to modern over-processed foods.

Consider making your own vinaigrettes. They are quick and easy. Use them on salads, drizzled on cooked or fresh vegetables, and as marinades for fish, chicken, or beef. The basic vinaigrette is three parts olive oil to one part vinegar. Add salt, pepper, and other spices at your whim. Blend with a whisk, or put all ingredients in a jar with a lid and shake it. Favor red wine or white wine vinegar over balsamic. Balsamic has the highest carb content of the vinegars. I suppose you could use apple cider vinegar, too. See chapter six for AMD vinaigrette in the Special Recipes section. Mix a batch and keep it in the refrigerator; it should be good for a week. You may be able to find a commercially prepared vinaigrette in the salad dressing section of the supermarket. If so, be sure the oil is predominantly olive oil (not very common) and that a serving (usually 2 tbsp or 30 ml) has no more than 2 g of carb.

5. DINING OUT

You'll be tempted to return to "normal" high-carb eating especially when you're away from your home's well-stocked cupboards and refrigerator. Be ready to deal with it.

One option is to take your food with you. For road trips, take nuts, fresh fruit, canned fish and meat, vegetables, an ice cooler stocked with condiments and your favorite no- or low-carb drinks. Don't forget disposable plates, utensils, and paper towels.

Buffets will have several low-carb paleo-friendly options for you.

Fast-food restaurants also offer several low-carb options. Order a burger and throw away the bun—or they may build the burger for you wrapped in lettuce (e.g., In N' Out and Carls Jr. in the U.S.). Fancy salads topped with chicken or beef are commonly available. Don't drown them with carb-heavy dressing. Nearly all fast-food restaurants provide nutritional analysis for menu items—ask for it if you aren't sure of the carb count.

6. CHEATING

Let's face it: sooner or later everybody cheats on diets.

It's easier to deal with the truth when you recognize the truth. It's not going to be the end of the world if you go "off plan" for one or two days a year and just eat like everyone else around you.

Of course, a meal or entire day with more than the usual amount of carb consumption can play havoc with blood sugar levels, which is a major potential problem. It's generally more of a problem in type 1 diabetes than type 2. (Prediabetics will have higher blood sugars, but rarely know it or suffer acute consequences.) If you have diabetes and plan on cheating now and then, plan ahead. Ask your doctor or diabetes nurse educator how you could handle temporarily higher blood sugars. Don't worry about being judged harshly; experienced clinicians know that diet compliance is never perfect. They won't go on the record and say "Go ahead and do it!" But they should help you minimize and deal with the consequences. Management options include: 1) taking additional insulin or other diabetic drugs, 2) adding some exercise—perhaps intense and prolonged—after the high-carb meal or item, 3) skipping the next meal, 4) eating the extra carbs before mid-afternoon so that physical activity later in the day will "burn up" the extra blood sugar, or 5) just living with temporarily high blood sugars.

Some diabetics decide it's just not worth the worry and hassle to plan for a cheat day or cheat meal. They just stay "on plan." More power to you! They often opt for low-carb versions of regular foods.

A more common issue is that someone has a craving for a particular food and can't live with the possibility of never eating it again. For instance, I love apple pie and Cinnabon cinnamon rolls; I might get depressed if I could never again have them. I don't have diabetes so my metabolism can handle the occasional sugar bomb. What I'll do, perhaps every couple months, is have the cinnamon roll (730 calories!) or a large serving of apple pie *instead of a meal.* Call it a "cheat meal." And I'll eat low-carb, maybe even lower than usual, for the remainder of that day. What about eating your usual three daily meals plus the cinnamon roll, and just burn off the extra calories with exercise? Sounds logical. But a 150-pound person (68 kg) would need to jump rope for four and a half hours to burn 730 calories. I won't do that, and you won't either.

Cheat days and cheat meals aren't an option for everyone. Think about alcoholics who have stopped drinking. Standard advice from addiction specialists, and I agree, is that alcoholics should never again drink alcohol. Not even a sip. Probably not even non-alcoholic "beer." That's because it's too tempting and could trigger a drinking binge, then uncontrollable drinking that's life-threatening. A few people are that way with carbohydrates. You could say they're addicted. They shouldn't have cheat days or cheat meals. Does this apply to you? Only you can answer that.

7. SWEET CRAVINGS

Sweet items on the Paleobetic Diet are fruits, and perhaps a little honey now and then. A teaspoon of honey has only 20 calories but 6 grams of digestible carbohydrate. Prevent high blood sugar spikes from fruits and honey by eating them with meals and in limited amounts.

If sweet cravings are your downfall, be aware that they tend to dissipate after several months of eating low-carb. It may take up to a year and it doesn't happen for everyone. You may also notice that certain foods, like nuts and carrots, start to taste sweeter than in the old days when you flooded your taste buds with sugar.

If your cravings persist and you can't resist them, your best option is artificial sweeteners, sometimes known as sugar substitutes. Examples are sucralose, aspartame, sorbitol, erythritol, and stevia. Several of these can be used in cooking and baking. They are all highly processed and not pure paleo. The stevia products may be closest to natural.

Online low-carb recipe repositories will have many sweet options. Or use off-the-shelf prepared items from grocery stores. Try sugar-free gelatin or sugar-free hard candy.

I have no objection if you wish to drink one or two diet soda pops a day. Water may be better for you.

8. HOLIDAYS

Holidays like Thanksgiving (in the U.S.) and Christmas present major temptations to folks trying to limit carb consumption and eat paleo-style. It's easier to stay "on plan" if you don't socialize much, but most of us visit relatives or others, and the temptation to eat like everyone else is great and often irresistible.

Sometimes people almost "force" carbs on you. Diabetics and prediabetics can just say, "No, thanks. My doctor has me on a special diet," and that should be the end of it. Others don't wish to reveal a medical condition and can say, "I'm fine, thank you. I just feel better if I eat a different way," or, "I'm fine, thank you. I'm not hungry right now." Still others are just totally honest and open and say, "No, thanks. That makes my blood sugar spike way too high." Practice your line of choice before you need it.

Another option is to cheat on the diet. See "Cheating" section above.

9. HUNGER

If you get hungry between meals, eat something that's either rich in protein or high in fat (or both) while being low-carb. Examples are meat, fish, eggs, avocado, nuts, or a leafy salad with high-fat dressing. Be careful with the nuts; easy to over-eat. If you just want something in your stomach, try a couple celery sticks (2 grams of net carbs, at most). Drink a glass of water.

Proteins in particular tend to be satiating, but on the other hand, tend to raise blood sugar more than fats do. In many folks, the protein effect on blood sugar is small, perhaps negligible. A large hard-boiled egg has 70 calories, of which 35% are from protein and 63% are from fat (I'm lumping cholesterol in with fats here). I've never known anyone to overeat and wreck his blood sugars with hard-boiled eggs.

A can of tuna, a chicken breast, or a couple hard-boiled eggs may not be your traditional snacks, but they aren't likely to blow your blood sugar control or weight management plan compared to a bag of corn chips or handful of cookies

10. RECORD-KEEPING

You can track your weight, blood sugars, and consumption of the major Paleobetic Diet food items with the "Paleobetic Diet Daily Log" available for free at:
https://paleodiabetic.files.wordpress.com/2014/04/paleobetic-diet-daily-log.pdf

If desired, you can pretty easily keep track of your daily consumption free online at a number of websites. One example is FitDay (http://fitday.com/). In addition to analyzing and recording what you eat, FitDay helps you readily track your weight and exercise and estimate calories burned exercising. It's definitely worth a look. At the end of the day, you'll get a comprehensive nutritional analysis of that day's consumption. And I mean comprehensive: overall percentages of calories from carbohydrate, protein, and fat, along with total calories and 40 or 50 vitamins, minerals, and other nutrients. Need to know how many digestible carb grams are in that apple you just ate? You'll find it at FitDay.

A similar website is SELF-NutritionData. The web address is http://nutritiondata.self.com/. First, register your free membership. Then go to the "My ND" section near the top of the page and click on "My Recipes." Make each of your days a single recipe with a title such as "Paleobetic Diet Day 1." Enter everything you eat in the course of a day. Remember to click "Save" before you leave that day's recipe. At the end of the day, choose the "Save and Analyze" button. You'll get a comprehensive nutritional analysis of that day's consumption. If you're going to do this for more than a couple days, use the "My Foods" feature and you'll end up saving time. A potential drawback, I suspect, is that no one has updated the food database for years.

Another good option for record-keeping is Calorie Count at http://caloriecount.about.com/. It's free, too.

Both Calorie Count and FitDay have active community forums for support and education. They are not designed specifically for diabetics, however.

An exercise like this—essentially a food diary—over four or five days is also helpful in figuring out why weight loss may have stalled or blood sugars are getting higher. Carb consumption and calories often creep up unnoticed, and at a certain point will sabotage the best-laid plans.

I bet there are smartphone apps for tracking food and exercise, but I'm not up-to-date on them.

11. WEIGHT-LOSS TIPS

Record-keeping is often the key to success. For options, see the section immediately preceding this.

Accountability is another key to success. Consider documenting your program and progress on a free website such as FitDay, SparkPeople, Calorie Count (http://caloriecount.about.com), or others. If your initiation to low-carb eating is a major undertaking (and it should be) consider blogging about your adventure on a free platform such as Wordpress or Blogger. Such a public commitment may be just what you need to keep you motivated.

Do you have a friend or spouse who wants to lose weight? Start the same program at the same time and support each other. That's built-in accountability.

If you tend to over-eat, floss and brush your teeth after you're full. You'll be less likely to go back for more anytime soon.

Eat at least two or three meals daily. Skipping meals may lead to uncontrollable overeating later on. On the other hand, ignore the diet gurus who say you must eat every two or three hours. That's codswallop.

Eat meals at a leisurely pace, chewing and enjoying each bite thoroughly before swallowing.

189

Plan to give yourself a specific reward for every 10 pounds (4.5 kg) of weight lost. You know what you like. Consider a weekend get-away, a trip to the beauty salon, jewelry, an evening at the theater, a professional massage, home entertainment equipment, new clothes, etc.

Carefully consider when would be a good time to start your new lifestyle. It should be a period of low or usual stress. Bad times would be Thanksgiving day, Christmas/New Years' holiday, the first day of a Caribbean cruise, and during a divorce.

If you know you've eaten enough at a meal to satisfy your nutritional requirements yet you still feel hungry, drink a large glass of water and wait a while.

Limit television to a maximum of a few hours a day.

Maintain a consistent eating pattern throughout the week and year.

Eat breakfast routinely.

Control emotional eating.

Weigh frequently: daily during active weight-loss efforts and during the first two months of your maintenance-of-weight-loss phase. After that, cut back to weekly weights if you want. Daily weights will remind you how hard you worked to achieve your goal.

Be aware that you might regain five or 10 pounds (2–4 kg) of fat now and then. You probably will. Don't freak out. It's human nature. You're not a failure; you're human. But draw the line and get back on the old weight-loss program for one or two months. Analyze and learn from the episode. Why did it happen? Slipping back into your old ways? Slacking off on exercise? Too many special occasion feasts or cheat days? Allowing junk food or non-essential carbs back into the house?

Learn which food item is your nemesis—the food that consistently torpedoes your resolve to eat right. For example, mine is anything sweet. Remember an old ad campaign for a potato chip: "Betcha can't eat just one!"? Well, I can't eat just one cookie. So I don't get started. I might eat one if it's the last one available. Or I satisfy my sweet craving with a diet soda, small piece of dark chocolate, or sugar-free gelatin. Just as a recovering alcoholic can't drink any alcohol, perhaps you should totally abstain from...? You know your own personal gastronomic Achilles heel. Or heels. Experiment with various strategies for vanquishing your nemesis.

If you're not losing excess weight as expected (about a pound or half a kilogram per week), you may benefit from eating just two meals a day. This will often turn on your cellular weight-loss machinery even when total calorie consumption doesn't seem much less than usual. The two meals to eat would be breakfast and a mid-afternoon meal (call it what you wish). The key is to not eat within six hours of bedtime. Of course, this trick could cause dangerous hypoglycemia if you're taking drugs with potential to cause low blood sugars, like insulin and sulfonylureas. Talk to your dietitian or physician before instituting a semi-radical diet change like this.

One of the bloggers I follow is James Fell. He says, "If you want to lose weight you need to cook. Period." James blogs at http://www.sixpackabs.com, with a focus on exercise and fitness.

Regular exercise is much more important for prevention of weight regain rather than for actually losing weight.

HOW TO OVERCOME A WEIGHT-LOSS STALL

It's common on any weight-loss program to be cruising along losing weight as promised, then suddenly the weight loss stops although you're still far from goal weight. This is the mysterious and infamous stall.

Once you know the cause for the stall, the way to break it becomes obvious. The most common reasons are:

- you're not really following the full program any more; you've drifted off the path, often unconsciously
- instead of eating just until you're full or satisfied, you're stuffing yourself
- you need to start or intensify an exercise program
- you've developed an interfering medical problem such as adrenal insufficiency (rare) or an underactive thyroid; see your doctor
- you're taking interfering medication such as a steroid; see your doctor
- your strength training program is building new muscle that masks ongoing loss of fat (not a problem!).

If you still can't figure out what's causing your stall, do a nutritional analysis of one weeks' worth of eating, with a focus on daily digestible carb (net carbs) and calorie totals. You can do this analysis online at places like FitDay (http://fitday.com/) or Calorie Count (http://caloriecount.about.com/).

What you do with your data depends on whether you're losing weight through portion control (usually reflecting calorie restriction) or carb counting. Most people lose weight with one of these two methods.

If you're a carb counter, you may find you've been sabotaged by "carb creep": excessive dietary carbs have insidiously invaded you. You need to cut back. Even if you're eating very-low-carb, it's still possible to have excess body fat, even gain new fat, if you eat too many calories from protein and fat. It's not easy, but it's possible.

Those who have followed a calorie-restriction weight loss model for a while may have become lax in their record-keeping. The stall is a result of simply eating too much. Call it "portion creep." You need to re-commit to observing portion sizes.

A final possible cause for a weight loss stall is that you just don't need as many calories as you once did. Think about this. Someone who weighs 300 lb (136 kg) is eating perhaps 3300 calories a day just to maintain a steady weight. He goes on a calorie-restricted diet (2800/day) and loses a pound (0.4 kg) a week. Eventually he's down to 210 lb (95.5 kg) but stalled, aiming for 180 lb (82 kg). The 210-lb body (95.5 kg) doesn't need 3300 calories a day to keep it alive and steady-state; it only needs 2800 and that's what it's getting. To restart the weight loss process, he has to reduce calories further, say down to 2300/day. This is not the "slowed down metabolism" we see with starvation or very-low-calorie diets. It's simply the result of getting rid of 90 pounds of fat (41 kg) that he no longer needs to feed.

12. Miscellanea

Use a food scale and measuring devices to improve your compliance with portion sizes, especially during the first month or two of the Paleobetic Diet. Thereafter you may be able to judge portion size by eye and feel.

An ounce (28 g) of nuts is about a quarter of a cup, or a heap of nuts in the palm of your hand, not covering your fingers.

Three ounces (85 g) of cooked meat or chicken is about the size of a deck of cards.

Fish and poultry may be a little more healthful for you than red meat.

Regular meat products may be a little healthier than processed meats like bacon, bologna and other luncheon meats, pre-cooked commercial sausages, etc.

I recommend at least two servings per week of cold-water fatty fish, for brain and heart health. Those fish include salmon, sardines, trout, herring, tuna, halibut, mackerel, and sea bass.

As long as a food is low-carb, don't go for the low-fat version. For instance, low-fat yogurt is over-loaded with carbohydrates (sugar) compared to the full-fat version. But yogurt isn't paleo anyway.

Tell your housemates you are on a special diet and ask for their support. You may also need to tell your co-workers and others with whom you spend significant time. If they care about you, they'll be careful not to tempt you off the diet.

Do your grocery shopping from a list.

If your blood sugars are running too high or if you're not losing excess weight as fast as expected, the problem may be that you've chosen the higher-carbohydrate options from the various food lists. For instance, the Paleobetic Diet includes 1–2 oz (30–60 g) nuts (primarily) or seeds daily. But one oz of cashews has eight g of digestible carb compared with only two g in almonds.

If you're blood sugars are running too high in the several hours after meals, consider reducing them with mealtime vinegar (56). Too high is glucose greater than 140 mg/dl or 7.8 mmol/l. The vinegar dose is two or three tsp (10–15 ml) of vinegar (5% acetic acid) in a cup (240 ml) of water, hot tea with lemon, or another appropriate beverage at mealtime.

13. SOCIAL ISSUES

GOING AGAINST THE GRAIN OF A CARB-CENTRIC CULTURE

There was a time in my life that I just loved whole grain bread, pizza, and pasta. I couldn't imagine life without them. As an experiment, I went an entire year eating low-carb, without whole grain bread, pizza, and pasta. At that point, I didn't miss them much at all. I realized I could easily have a happy, healthy, fulfilling, life without whole grain bread, pizza, and pasta. If you told me I had a medical condition that would worsen if I ate them, I could easily live without them and not complain.

During that same experimental year, I cut way back on my consumption of sweet fruits, starchy vegetables, and sweets (cookies, cakes, candy bars, pies). After the year was up, I didn't miss the sweet fruits and starchy vegetables, although I did miss my sweet things. I could see living the rest of my life without sweet fruits and starchy vegetables. Giving up apple pie and Cinnabon cinnamon rolls would be tougher.

That's just my experience, but I'm not alone. I wouldn't ask you to give up many of your beloved carbohydrates if I didn't know it was possible, and that others had done it successfully. The trade-offs for many of us will be improved health and slimmer waistlines.

The odd thing about the Paleobetic Diet is that it goes against the grain (pun intended) of the Western food culture that prominently features carbohydrates. Anyone following the diet is immediately in a strange position, surrounded continuously with opportunities and inducements to consume carbs. Especially nutrient-depleted, highly refined carbs such as white bread, sugar, flour, fruit juice, potato and corn chips, high fructose corn syrup, and soda pop.

It's difficult to be immersed in such a culture, especially for a diabetic or prediabetic who may have lived happily and healthfully in that society for 40 years before diagnosis. Old habits are hard to break. Food preferences are deeply ingrained from an early age.

The only way I know to counteract that cultural pull is to take to heart the medical consequences of continued participation in that poisonous environment. Frankly, it's not going to matter much if your blood sugar today is 211 mg/dl versus 93 mg/dl (11.7 mmol/l versus 5.2 mmol/l). But if that difference is sustained over years, you're putting yourself at risk for all the usual diabetic complications that would degrade the quality and duration of your life.

How do you motivate someone today to make a radical change in behavior that may not have a pay-off for another decade or more? Education is the only tactic I know that works consistently. People are more receptive when they're hospitalized with diabetic symptoms and blood sugars are 450 mg/dl (25 mmol/l). Even then change is often a struggle.

Millions of people with normal carbohydrate metabolism have used very-low-carb eating as a way to lose excess weight and keep it off. It's a little easier for diabetics and prediabetics to stick with it in light of the potential health and longevity benefits. Low-carbing for them is not so much a lifestyle choice as it is a medical necessity.

Low-carb eating increasingly will be seen as viable and healthful as news of recent scientific developments becomes mainstream. Low-carbing will be easier to maintain then, diabetic or not.

The Paleobetic Diet is a radical departure from the way most people are used to eating. Too radical, perhaps, for a majority of diabetics and prediabetics to sustain for a lifetime. I can't guarantee a diabetic will live longer or have fewer complications by following it. I can guarantee I'd follow it or another major carbohydrate-restricted diet if I had diabetes or prediabetes myself. For most followers, it will result in blood sugar levels much closer to the normal range, compared to the way most people with diabetes eat in 2015.

But enough philosophizing.

ONLINE SUPPORT

If you feel lonely and odd eating low-carb, you will find copious online support at the Low Carb Friends message boards (http://lowcarbfriends.com/) and Active Low-Carbers Forum (http://forum.lowcarber.org/). There are plenty of low-carbers also on the forums at FitDay, Spark-People, and 3FatChicks. None of these sites are specifically and exclusively for paleo-style low-carbers, however.

PARTIES AND HOLIDAY MEALS

In general, I think it's a good idea to let those around you know that you're eating low-carb paleo. I understand you may have good reasons to keep it a secret, however. If you're not in charge of the food, let the host know you'll be focusing on meat, chicken, eggs, fish, fruit, nuts, and low-carb vegetables. The meats are usually main courses anyway. You'll simply not be eating many of the side dishes like bread, potatoes, corn, peas, and desserts. If you're the host, I'm sure you'll want to provide your guests—especially children—with the usual high-carb fare. With some experience, you could serve adults a delicious low-carb paleo feast without their awareness.

If the host is a vegetarian or vegan serving his usual cuisine, you may have fewer options. If available, you may well be satisfied with low-carb vegetables, nuts, and fruit. Think about eating before the event, and then just eat a little to be cordial.

11
Exercise

S. Boyd Eaton and Stanley Eaton have estimated late Stone Age activity levels based on recent hunter-gatherer societies and skeletal remains from 50,000 to 20,000 years ago (35). Our bones reflect how much work we ask them to do. Heavy physical work loads over time lead to thicker, stronger bones, even changing the cross-sectional shape of long bones from round to oval.

From a diabetes viewpoint, the scientists expect that our prehistoric ancestors had excellent insulin sensitivity in view of their relatively larger muscle mass and high activity levels. They would have been less prone to develop type 2 diabetes.

The habitual high levels of physical activity of our ancestors put them in the same class as today's elite cross-training athletes. Hunting, foraging, avoiding predators, building shelter, and hauling water were labor-intensive compared to our current lifestyles.

The Eatons suggest that replication of the Paleolithic activity level would require we exercise about an hour a day, not the 30 minutes recommended by many public health authorities. The hour a day equates to about 490 calories or 2.1 MJ. For a 150-pound person (62 kg) to burn 490 calories in exercise would require five hours of singles tennis, four hours of jogging, or five hours of brisk walking (4 mph). Heavier folks burn more calories per hour for the same activities.

If you're buying into the whole Paleolithic lifestyle re-creation, you need to start exercising more! But I don't think that much exercise is necessary for optimal health.

GENERAL EXERCISE BENEFITS

Regular physical activity postpones death, mostly by its effect on cancer, heart attacks, and strokes.

Peak aerobic power (or fitness) naturally diminishes by 50 percent between young adulthood and age 65. Regular exercise increases fitness (aerobic power) by 15–20 percent in middle-aged and older men and women, the equivalent of a 10–20 year reduction in biological age!

Additional benefits of exercise include: 1) enhanced immune function, 2) stronger bones, 3) preservation and improvement of flexibility, 4) lower blood pressure by 8–10 points, 5) diminished premenstrual bloating, breast tenderness, and mood changes, 6) reduced incidence of dementia, 7) less trouble with constipation, 7) better ability to handle stress, 8) less trouble with insomnia, 9) improved self-esteem, 10) enhanced sense of well-being, with less anxiety and depression, 11) higher perceived level of energy, and 12) prevention of weight regain.

EXERCISE EFFECT ON DIABETES

Eighty-five percent of type 2 diabetics are overweight or obese. It's not just a random association. Obesity contributes to many cases of type 2 diabetes, particularly in those predisposed by heredity. Insulin is the key that allows bloodstream glucose into cells for utilization as energy, thus keeping blood sugar from reaching dangerously high levels. Overweight and obese bodies produce plenty of insulin, often more than average. The problem in many type 2 diabetics is that the cells are no longer sensitive to insulin's effect. (We see this in some overweight and obese type 1 patients as well.) Weight loss and exercise independently return insulin sensitivity towards normal. Many diabetics can improve their condition through sensible exercise and weight management.

Muscles doing prolonged exercise soak up sugar from the blood stream to use as an energy source, a process occurring independent of insulin's effect. On the other hand, blood sugar may rise early in the course of an exercise session.

EXERCISE RECOMMENDATIONS

Please note that you don't have to run marathons (26.2 miles or 42.16 km) or compete in the Ironman Triathlon to earn the health benefits of exercise. However, if health promotion and disease prevention are your goals, plan on a lifetime commitment to regular physical activity.

For the general public, the U.S. Centers for Disease Control and Prevention recommends at least 150 minutes per week of moderate-intensity aerobic activity (e.g., brisk walking) and muscle-strengthening activity at least twice a week, OR 75 minutes per week of vigorous-intensity aerobic activity (e.g., running or jogging) plus muscle-strengthening activity at least twice a week. The muscle-strengthening activity should work all the major muscle groups: legs, hips, back, abdomen, chest, shoulders, arms.

The American Diabetes Association's Standards of Care in Diabetes–2015 state that "Adults with diabetes should be advised to perform at least 150 min/week of moderate-intensity aerobic physical activity (50–70% of maximum heart rate), spread over at least 3 days/week with no more than two consecutive days without exercise." Unless contraindicated, adults with type 2 diabetes should perform resistance training at least twice per week. Everybody, diabetes or not, should reduce sedentary time, particularly by breaking up extended sitting episodes longer than 90 minutes.

STRENGTH TRAINING

What's strength training? It's also called muscle-strengthening activity, resistance training, weight training, and resistance exercise. Examples include lifting weights, work with resistance bands, digging, shoveling, yoga, push-ups, chin-ups, and other exercises that use your body weight or other loads for resistance.

Strength training just twice a week increases your strength and endurance, allows you to sculpt your body to an extent, and counteracts the loss of lean body mass (muscle) so often seen during efforts to lose excess weight. It also helps maintain your functional abilities as you age. For example, it's a major chore for many 80-year-olds to climb a flight of stairs, carry in a bag of groceries from the car, or vacuum a house. Strength training helps maintain these abilities that youngsters take for granted.

According to the U.S. Centers for Disease Control and Prevention: "To gain health benefits, muscle-strengthening activities need to be done to the point where it's hard for you to do another repetition without help. A repetition is one complete movement of an activity, like lifting a weight or doing a sit-up. Try to do 8–12 repetitions per activity that count as 1 set. Try to do at least 1 set of muscle-strengthening activities, but to gain even more benefits, do 2 or 3 sets."

If this is starting to sound like Greek to you, consider instruction by a personal trainer at a local gym or health club. That's a good investment for anyone unfamiliar with strength training, in view of its great benefits and the potential harm or waste of time from doing it wrong. Alternatives to a personal trainer would be help from an experienced friend, instructional DVDs, or even YouTube videos. If you're determined to go it alone, Internet resources may help (36), but be careful.

Current strength training techniques are much different than what you remember from high school 30 years ago—modern methods are better. Some of the latest research suggests that strength training may be even more beneficial than aerobic exercise.

AEROBIC ACTIVITY

What's aerobic activity? Just about anything that
mostly makes you huff and puff. In other words, get
short of breath to some degree. Examples are brisk
walking, swimming, golf (pulling a cart or carrying
clubs), lawn work, painting, home repair, racket
sports and table tennis, house cleaning, leisurely
canoeing, jogging, bicycling, jumping rope, and ski-
ing. The possibilities are endless. A leisurely stroll
in the shopping mall doesn't qualify, unless that
makes you short of breath. Don't laugh: that's a
workout for many who are obese and out of shape.

But which aerobic physical activity is best? Ideally,
it's an activity that's pleasant for you. If not outright
fun, it should be often enjoyable and always tolerable.

Your exercise of choice should also be available
year-round, affordable, safe, and utilize large muscle groups. The greater mass and number of muscles used, the more calories you will burn, which is
important if you're trying to lose weight or prevent
gain. Compare tennis playing with sitting in a chair
squeezing a tennis ball repetitively. The tennis player burns calories much faster. Your largest muscles
are in your legs, so consider walking, biking, many
team sports, ski machines, jogging, treadmill,
swimming, water aerobics, stationary cycling, stair-
steppers, tennis, volleyball, roller-skating, rowing,
jumping rope, and yard work.
Walking is "just what the doctor ordered" for many
people. It's readily available, affordable, usually
safe, and requires little instruction. If it's too hot,
too cold, or rainy outside, you can do it in a mall,
gymnasium, or health club.

EXERCISE IS NOT FUN

Wait, what? I've written above that the physical activity you choose should be pleasant if not outright enjoyable. Tolerable at a minimum. That's standard advice you'll read everywhere. However, Ken Hutchins wrote an eye-opening essay ("Exercise vs Recreation") with the main point being, exercise isn't supposed to be fun (37). "If it is, then you should suspect that something is wrong," Hutchins wrote. Recreation is fun; exercise isn't. To gain the benefits of exercise, it has to be physically demanding. Playing on a volleyball team, soccer team, or softball team is fun physical activity, but it's not necessarily demanding. Walking in the neighborhood 30 minutes a day may be enjoyable, but isn't necessarily demanding.

When I was a young man in my 30s, I was jogging 20 miles a week and ran a couple marathons. I enjoyed it and didn't do much else for exercise or overall fitness. I thought I was in pretty good shape. You can get away with that when you're 35, but not when you're 50. At 60 now, I can't think of any single recreational activity that can help me maintain the overall strength, functionality, and injury resistance I want and need as I age.

I've come to view exercise as a chore, like flossing/brushing teeth, changing the oil in my car, and sleeping when I'd rather not. I've got my current exercise chore whittled down to 45 minutes twice a week. It's demanding and not enjoyable.

Hutchins wrote, "Do not try to make exercise enjoyable." Getting your teeth cleaned isn't supposed to be fun, either. Once I got that through my thick skull, it made it easier for me to slog through my twice weekly workouts.

Another Hutchins quote: "We accept that both exercise and recreation are important in the overall scheme of fitness, and they overlap to a great degree. But to reap maximum benefits of both or either they must first be well-defined and then be segregated in practice." And finally, "Perhaps the most destructive as well as most misunderstood concept in fitness today among researchers, the commercial health facilities, and the general public alike is the confusion of exercise and recreation."

MEDICAL CLEARANCE

To protect you from injury, I recommend that you obtain "medical clearance" from a personal physician before starting an exercise program. A physician is in the best position to determine if your plans are safe for you, thereby avoiding complications such as injury and death. Nevertheless, most adults can start a moderate-intensity exercise program with little risk. An example of moderate intensity would be walking briskly (3–4 mph or 4.8–6.4 km/h) for 30 minutes daily.

Men over 40 and women over 50 who anticipate a more vigorous program should consult a physician to ensure safety. The physician may well recommend diagnostic blood work, an electrocardiogram (heart electrical tracing), and an exercise stress test (often on a treadmill). The goal is not to generate fees for the doctor, but to find the occasional person for whom exercise will be dangerous, if not fatal. Those who drop dead at the start of a vigorous exercise program often have an undiagnosed heart condition, such as blockages in the arteries that supply the heart muscle. The doctor will also look for other dangerous undiagnosed "silent" conditions, such as leaky heart valves, hereditary heart conditions, aneurysms, extremely high blood pressure, and severe diabetes.

The American Diabetes Association's Standards of Care–2015 state that routine testing of all diabetics for heart artery blockages before an exercise program is not recommended; the doctor should use judgment case-by-case. Many diabetics (and their doctors) are unaware that they already have "silent" coronary artery disease (CAD). CAD is defined by blocked or clogged heart arteries, which reduce the blood flow to the hard-working heart muscle. Your heart pumps 100,000 times a day, every day, for years without rest. CAD raises the odds of fainting, heart attack, or sudden death during strenuous exercise.

I tend to favor a cardiac stress test (or the equivalent) to all diabetics prior to moderate or vigorous exercise programs, particularly if over 40 years old. The idea is that CAD can thus be diagnosed and treated before complications arise. Ask your personal physician for her opinion.

Regardless of age and diabetes, other folks who may benefit from a medical consultation before starting an exercise program include those with known high blood pressure, high cholesterol, joint problems (e.g., arthritis, degenerated discs), neurologic problems, poor circulation, lung disease, or any other significant chronic medical condition. Also be sure to check with a doctor first if you've been experiencing chest pains, palpitations, dizziness, fainting spells, headaches, frequent urination, or any unusual symptoms (particularly during exertion).

Physicians, physiatrists, physical therapists, and exercise physiologists can also be helpful in the design of a safe, effective exercise program for those with established chronic medical conditions.

BASELINE AND PERIODIC MEASUREMENTS

Before beginning or modifying a fitness program, it's interesting and edifying to take some baseline physical measurements. Re-measure periodically. That way you'll know whether you're making progress, holding steady, or regressing. Seeing improvement in the numbers also helps to maintain motivation. Not taking measurements would be like starting a weight loss program without a baseline and subsequent weights. You may appreciate an assistant to help you measure some of these.

WHAT TO MEASURE

Minimal

Weight
Blood pressure
Waist circumference (I prefer measuring in supine position)
Maximum number of consecutive pull-ups or chin-ups
Maximum number of consecutive push-ups
Maximum number of consecutive sit-ups
Walk or run one mile as fast as you can (time it)

Extra Credit or OCD Folks

Height
Body mass index
Mid-arm circumference, both arms, hanging relaxed at your sides

Maximal calf circumference, both calves, while standing at ease

Resting heart rate (first thing in the AM before getting out of bed)

Maximum vertical jump (stand by a tall wall then jump and reach up as high as you can with one arm, noting the highest point above ground your fingers can reach)

Can you touch your toes? Stand up straight, locking knees in extension, then bend over at your waist and touch your toes with your fingertips. If you can touch toes, can you flatten your palms against the floor? If you can't reach your toes, measure the distance from your fingertips to the floor.

Optional Blood Work for Special Situations

Fasting blood sugar, hemoglobin A1c, cholesterol, HDL-cholesterol, LDL-cholesterol, and trigylcerides. If coronary artery disease (e.g., heart attacks) runs in your family, consider checking your LDL-particle number (LDL-P), apolipoprotein B (apoB), and lipoprotein(a) since these may be better predictors of risk than the various cholesterol levels.

WHAT TO EXPECT GOING FORWARD

Record and retain your numbers. Re-test some or all of these periodically. If you're in fairly poor condition at the outset, you'll see some improved physical performance numbers after a couple or three weeks of a good exercise program. It takes months to build significant muscle mass; you'll see improved strength and endurance before mass.

The particular aspects of fitness these measure are strength and endurance in major muscle groups, cardiovascular and pulmonary endurance, a little flexibility, and a hint of body composition.

It will take several months to see significant changes in the blood tests.

There's no consensus as to what constitutes an adequate level of fitness. Some would say it's the level that will allow you to do the things in life you want to do, with a reasonable level of comfort. For instance, if you want to climb K2 (28,251 feet or 8611 meters above sea level), you'll need an incredibly high level of fitness. On the other hand, if you're a desk jockey and spend all your free time watching YouTube, you don't need much fitness. The level required for that life won't get you the overall health benefits of exercise discussed at the start of the chapter. What I've settled on for myself is to be able to pass the U.S. Army physical fitness requirements. They're based on age and sex. All army soldiers have to pass the test every six months. It simply involves how many consecutive push-ups you can do, how many consecutive sit-ups you can do, and how long does it take you to run or walk two miles. See how you stack up here: http://usmilitary.about.com/od/army/a/afpt.htm

EXERCISE AND THE DIABETIC

People with diabetes may have specific problem areas related to exercise.

DIABETIC RETINOPATHY

Retinopathy, an eye disease caused by diabetes, increases risk of retinal detachment and bleeding into the eyeball called vitreous hemorrhage. These can cause blindness. Vigorous aerobic or resistance training may increase the odds of these serious eye complications. Patients with retinopathy may not be able to safely participate. If you have any degree of retinopathy, avoid the straining and breath-holding that is so often done during weightlifting or other forms of resistance exercise. Vigorous aerobic exercise may also pose a risk. By all means, check with your ophthalmologist first. You don't want to experiment with your eyes.

DIABETIC FEET AND PERIPHERAL NEUROPATHY

Diabetics are prone to foot ulcers, infections, and ingrown toenails, especially if peripheral neuropathy (numbness or loss of sensation) is present. Proper foot care, including frequent inspection, is more important than usual if a diabetic exercises with his feet. Daily inspection should include the soles and in-between the toes, looking for blisters, redness, calluses, cracks, scrapes, or breaks in the skin. See your physician or podiatrist for any abnormalities. Proper footwear is important (for example, don't crowd your toes). Dry feet should be treated with a moisturizer regularly. In cases of severe peripheral neuropathy, non-weight-bearing exercise (e.g., swimming or cycling) may be preferable. Discuss with your physician or podiatrist.

HYPOGLYCEMIA

Low blood sugars are a risk during exercise if you take diabetic medications in the following classes: insulins, sulfonylureas, meglitinides, and possibly thiazolidinediones and bromocriptine. Hypoglycemia is very uncommon with thiazolidinediones. Bromocriptine is so new (for diabetes) that we have little experience with it; hypoglycemia is probably rare or non-existent.

Diabetics and prediabetics treated with diet alone or other medications rarely have trouble with hypoglycemia during exercise.

Always check your blood sugar before an exercise session if you are at risk for hypoglycemia. Always have glucose tablets, such as Dextrotabs, available if you are at risk for hypoglycemia. Hold off on your exercise if your blood sugar is over 200 mg/dl (11.1 mmol/l) and you don't feel well, because exercise has the potential to raise blood sugar even further early in the course of an exercise session. As the session continues, active muscles may soak up bloodstream glucose as an energy source, leaving less circulating glucose available for other tissues such as your brain. Vigorous exercise can reduce blood sugar levels below 60 mg/dl (3.33 mmol/l), although it's rarely a problem in non-diabetics.

The degree of glucose removal from the bloodstream by exercising muscles depends on how much muscle tissue is working, and how hard. Vigorous exercise by several large muscles will remove more glucose. Compare a long rowing race to a slow stroll around the neighborhood. The rower is strenuously using large muscles in the legs, arms, and back. The rower will pull much more glucose out of circulation. Of course, other metabolic processes are working to put more glucose into circulation as exercising muscles remove it. Carbohydrate consumption and diabetic medications are going to affect this balance one way or the other.

If you are at risk for hypoglycemia, check your blood sugar before your exercise session. If under 90 mg/dl (5.0 mmol/l), eat a meal or chew some glucose tablets to prevent exercise-induced hypoglycemia. Re-test your blood sugar 30–60 minutes later, before you exercise, to be sure it's over 90 mg/dl (5.0 mmol/l). The peak effect of the glucose tablets will be 30–60 minutes later. If the exercise session is long or strenuous, you may need to chew glucose tablets every 15–30 minutes. If you don't have glucose tablets, keep a carbohydrate source with you or nearby in case you develop hypoglycemia during exercise.

Re-check your blood sugar 30–60 minutes after exercise since it may tend to go too low.

If you are at risk of hypoglycemia and performing moderately vigorous or strenuous exercise, you may need to check your blood sugar every 15–30 minutes during exercise sessions until you have established a predictable pattern. Reduce the frequency once you're convinced that hypoglycemia won't occur. Return to frequent blood sugar checks when your diet or exercise routine changes.

These general guidelines don't apply across the board to each and every diabetic. Our metabolisms are all different. The best way to see what effect diet and exercise will have on your glucose levels is to monitor them with your home glucose measuring device, especially if you are new to exercise or you work out vigorously. You can pause during your exercise routine and check a glucose level, particularly if you don't feel well.

Carbohydrate or calorie restriction combined with a moderately strenuous or vigorous exercise program may necessitate a 50 percent or more reduction in your insulin, sulfonylurea, or meglitinide. Or the dosage may need to be reduced only on days of heavy workouts. Again, enlist the help of your personal physician, dietitian, diabetes nurse educator, and home glucose monitor.

Finally, insulin users should be aware that insulin injected over muscles that are about to be exercised may get faster absorption into the bloodstream. Blood sugar may then fall rapidly and too low. For example, injecting into the thigh and then going for a run may cause a more pronounced insulin effect compared to injection into the abdomen or arm.

AUTONOMIC NEUROPATHY

This issue is pretty technical and pertains to function of automatic, unconscious body functions controlled by nerves. These reflexes can be abnormal, particularly in someone who's had diabetes for many years, and are called autonomic neuropathy. Take your heart rate, for example. It's there all the time, you don't have to think about it. If you run to catch a bus or climb two flights of stairs, your heart rate increases automatically to supply more blood to exercising muscles. If that automatic reflex doesn't work properly, exercise is more dangerous, possibly leading to passing out, dizziness, and poor exercise tolerance. Other automatic nerve systems control our body temperature regulation (exercise may overheat you), stomach emptying (your blood sugar may go too low), and blood pressure (it could drop too low). Only your doctor can tell for sure if you have autonomic neuropathy.

DIABETIC KIDNEY DISEASE

Good news: no need for specific exercise precautions.

IF YOU ARE MARKEDLY OBESE

The more overweight you are, the harder it will be to exercise. At some point even light exercise becomes impossible. Average-height women tipping the scales at about 280 pounds (127 kg) and men at 360 pounds (164 kg) aren't going to be able to jog around the block, much less run a marathon. These weights are 100 percent over ideal or healthy levels. An actual "exercise program" probably won't be possible until some weight is lost simply through very-low-carb eating, calorie restriction, or bariatric surgery. The initial exercise goal for you may just be to get moving through activities of daily living and perhaps brief walks and calisthenics while sitting in a chair.

Markedly obese people who aren't up to the aforementioned extreme weights can usually tolerate a low-intensity physical activity program. At 50 percent over ideal weight, an average-height woman of 210 pounds (95 kg) is carrying 70 excess pounds (32 kg) of fat. Her male counter-part lugs around 90 pounds (41 kg) of unnecessary fat. This weight burden causes dramatic breathlessness and fatigue upon exertion, and makes the joints and muscles more susceptible to aching and injury. If you're skinny, just imagine trying to walk or run a mile carrying a standard five-gallon (19 liter) water cooler bottle, which weighs only 43 pounds (19.5 kg) when full. The burden of excess fat makes it quite difficult to exercise.

If you're markedly obese, several tricks will enhance your exercise success. I want you to avoid injury, frustration, and burn out. Start with light activity for only 10 or 15 minutes, gradually increase session length (e.g., by two to four minutes every two to four weeks) and increase exercise intensity only after several months. Your joints and muscles may appreciate easy, low-impact exercises such as stationary cycling, walking, swimming, and pool calisthenics/water aerobics. You may also benefit from the advice of a personal fitness trainer arranged through a health club, gym, or YMCA/YWCA. Check out several health clubs before you join. Some of them are primarily meat markets for beautiful slender yuppies. You may feel more comfortable in a gym that welcomes and caters to overweight people. Many hospitals offer fitness centers designed with obese orthopedic, heart, and diabetic patients in mind.

EXERCISE WITH JOINT AND BACK PAIN

Painful lower limb joints and chronic or recurrent back pain are exercise barriers to many people. Those affected should consult a physician for a diagnosis, treatment, and advice on appropriate physical activity. If the physician isn't sure about an exercise prescription, consultation with an orthopedist, physiatrist, or physical therapist should be helpful. Generally, weight-bearing on bad joints should be minimized by doing pool calisthenics, stationary cycling, swimming, etc. Use your imagination. Particularly bothersome joints may not tolerate exercise, if ever, until weight is lost by some other method. Light to moderate exercise actually reduces the pain and disability of knee degenerative arthritis. The effect is modest and comes with a small risk of injury such as bone fracture, cartilage tears, arthritis flare, and soft tissue strain.

SUMMARY

All I'm asking you to do is aerobic activity, such as walk briskly (3–4 mph or 4.8–6.4 km/h) for 30 minutes most days of the week, and do some muscle-strengthening exercises two or three times a week. These recommendations are also consistent with the American Diabetes Association's Standards of Care—2015. This amount of exercise will get you most of the documented health benefits.

I'm developing an exercise program that requires only 35 minutes twice a week, but it's not ready for prime time. Follow my progress at my Advanced Mediterranean Life blog:
http://advancedmediterranean.com.

Let me be clear. Exercise is not important because it burns calories! Exercise without calorie restriction is a remarkably ineffective weight loss intervention, because it usually makes us hungry enough to replace the calories we burn. Exercise is important because it restores your ability to oxidize fat—both when fasting and after meals.

—J. Stanton at Gnolls.org

The below-parallel squat is the best exercise in the entire catalog for whole-body strength, power, balance, coordination, bone density, joint integrity, and mental toughness—good things to develop if you don't have them.

—Mark Rippetoe, author of *Starting Strength*

12
Normal Blood Sugars and Treatment Goals

Physicians focus so much on disease that we sometimes lose sight of what's healthy and normal. For instance, the American Diabetes Association defines "tight control" of diabetes to include sugar levels as high as 179 mg/dl (9.94 mmol/l) when measured two hours after a meal. In contrast, young adults without diabetes two hours after a meal are usually in the range of 90 to 110 mg/dl (5.0–6.1 mmol/l).

WHAT IS A NORMAL BLOOD SUGAR LEVEL?

The following numbers refer to average blood sugar (glucose) levels in venous plasma, obtained by sticking a needle into a vein, and measured in a lab. Portable home glucose meters measure sugar in capillary whole blood, as opposed to venous plasma. Many meters in 2015—but not all—are calibrated to compare directly to venous plasma levels.

AVERAGE BLOOD SUGAR VALUES BEFORE AND AFTER A MEAL:

Fasting blood sugar after a night of sleep and before
    breakfast: 85 mg/dl (4.72 mmol/l)
One hour after a meal: 110 mg/dl (6.11 mmol/l)
Two hours after a meal: 95 mg/dl (5.28 mmol/l)
Five hours after a meal: 85 mg/dl (4.72 mmol/l)

(These glucose values assume a meal deriving 50–55% of its calories from carbohydrate—a typical carbohydrate percentage.)

RANGES OF BLOOD SUGAR FOR YOUNG HEALTHY NON-DIABETIC ADULTS:

Fasting blood sugar: 70–90 mg/dl (3.9–5.0 mmol/l)
One hour after a typical meal: 90–125 mg/dl (5.0–
    6.94 mmol/l)
Two hours after a typical meal: 90–110 mg/dl (5.0–
    6.1 mmol/l)
Five hours after a typical meal: 70–90 mg/dl (3.9–
    5.0 mmol/l)

BLOOD SUGAR AND HEMOGLOBIN A1C GOALS DURING TREATMENT FOR DIABETES

THE AMERICAN DIABETES ASSOCIATION (IN 2015) RECOMMENDS:

Fasting blood glucose: 80–130 mg/dl (4.4–7.2
    mmol/l)

Peak postprandial (1–2 hours after start of meal) capillary plasma glucose: under 180 mg/dl (under 10 mmol/l)

Hemoglobin A1c: under 7%. Lower values (under 6.5%) might be suggested for selected individuals.

Note that a hemoglobin A1c of 7% is equivalent to average blood sugar levels of 154 mg/dl (8.6 mmol/l). Hemogobin A1c of 6% equals, roughly, average blood sugar levels of 126 mg/dl (7.0 mmol/l). But remember, healthy non-diabetics spend most of their day under 100 mg/dl (5.56 mmol/l) and have hemoglobin A1c's around 5%.

THE 2013 GUIDELINES OF THE AMERICAN ASSOCIATION OF CLINICAL ENDOCRINOLOGISTS FOCUS ON HEMOGLOBIN A1C RATHER THAN BLOOD SUGARS:

Hemoglobin A1c: 6.5% or less for otherwise healthy people who are also at low risk for hypoglycemia. For those with one or more significant illnesses and at risk for hypoglycemia, hemoglobin A1c over 6.5% is fine. In other words, the target is individualized and based on a number of factors. Hemoglobin A1c of 6.5% equates to blood sugars that average 140 mg/dl (7.8 mmol/l).

IN 2011, THE AACE RECOMMENDED BLOOD SUGAR GOALS

Fasting Blood Sugar: under 110 mg/dl (6.1 mmol/l)
Two Hours After a Meal: under 140 mg/dl (7.78 mmol/l)

Diabetes experts actively debate how tightly we should control blood sugar levels. For instance, Dr.

Richard K. Bernstein—a diabetologist and type 1 diabetic himself—recommends keeping blood sugar levels under 90 mg/dl (5.0 mmol/l) almost all the time. If it exceeds 95 mg/dl (5.3 mmol/l) after a meal, then a change in medication or meal is in order, he says.

The ADA reminds clinicians, and I'm sure the AACE guys agree, that diabetes control goals should be individualized, based on age and life expectancy of the patient, duration of diabetes, other diseases that are present, individual patient preferences, and whether the patient is able to easily recognize and deal with hypoglycemia. I agree completely. For instance, there's not much reason to aim for blood sugars of 100 mg/dl (5.56 mmol/l) in a 79-year-old expected to die of lung cancer in four months. The goal for him is comfort and symptom relief, even if sugars are 220 mg/dl (12.2 mmol/l) and hemoglobin A1c is 9.5%.

Here's the over-simplified "tight control" debate. On one hand, tight control helps prevent and may reverse some of the devastating consequences of diabetes, such as nerve damage, eye damage, and kidney disease. On the other hand, tight control in diabetics on insulin and certain other diabetic medications may raise the risk of life-threatening hypoglycemia and may shorten lifespan in other ways.

BLOOD SUGAR GOALS FOR MY PERSONAL DIABETIC AND PREDIABETIC PATIENTS

Ideally, in general, I like to see normal glucose levels before and after meals, with normal hemoglobin A1c (see normal levels above). Realistically, these are acceptable fall-back positions:

Fasting Blood Sugar: under 100 mg/dl (5.56

mmol/l)
One Hour After Meals: under 150 mg/dl (8.33
    mmol/l)
Two Hours After Meals: under 130 mg/dl
    (7.22mmol/l)
Hemoglobin A1c: 6% or less

Undoubtedly, these goals are not acceptable or achievable by everyone with diabetes.

Treatment options for those not at goal include diet modification, loss of excess weight, exercise, and medication adjustments. Future studies may prove that such strict goals are not necessary to avoid the complications and premature death suffered by some diabetics. Tight control may be less important for elderly diabetics over 65–70. But for now, if I were a young or middle-aged diabetic I'd shoot for the goals above.

...built into our genes is a blueprint for optimal nutrition—a plan that spells out the foods that make us healthy, lean, and fit. Whether you believe the architect of that blueprint is God, or God acting throughout evolution by natural selection, or by evolution alone, the end result is still the same: We need to give our bodies the foods we were originally designed to eat.

—Loren Cordain in *The Paleo Diet*

13
Long-Term Maintenance

As a diabetic or prediabetic trying to get and stay healthy, you need at least two other players on your healthcare team: a physician and a registered dietitian. Additionally, diabetes nurse educators can be quite helpful in teaching you to manage your condition. Other care team members may include physician assistants, nurse practitioners, pharmacists, and nutritionists.

Dietitians are particularly helpful consultants when diabetes is first diagnosed and periodically thereafter to answer food questions, check on compliance with diet recommendations, and to review new dietary guidelines. Unfortunately, a majority of dietitians still believe the outdated idea that high-carbohydrate eating is healthy for diabetics and others who have demonstrable difficulty processing carbs. Be sure the dietitian you choose supports a low-carb way of eating.

Most primary care physicians such as family physicians and internists are well-trained to co-manage diabetes with you. I chose the word "co-manage" carefully. It's not like you have appendicitis and can turn over all management to a surgeon. With diabetes, you have to do more work than your physician. Your doctor will review your home glucose records, adjust medications, periodically examine you, and check blood work. You need a doctor who will support, or at least tolerate, your low-carb paleo way of eating.

An endocrinologist can be an invaluable team member, either as your main treating physician or as a consultant to your primary care physician. You should definitely see one if you are not close to the standard treatment goals after working with your primary care physician.

PERIODIC TESTS, TREATMENTS, AND GOALS

The American Diabetes Association (ADA) recommends the following items be done yearly (except as noted) in non-pregnant adults with diabetes. Incidentally, I don't necessarily agree with all ADA guidelines. ADA guidelines with supporting documentation are available free on the Internet (search for "Standards of Medical Care in Diabetes—2015"):

- Lipid profile (every year or two if results are fine and stable)
- Comprehensive foot exam
- Screening tests for distal symmetric polyneuropathy, such as pinprick, vibration,

monofilament pressure sense, and ankle reflexes
- Serum creatinine and estimate of glomerular filtration rate
- Test for albumin in the urine, such as measurement of albumin-to-creatinine ratio in a random spot urine specimen
- Comprehensive eye exam by an ophthalmologist (if exam is normal, every two years is acceptable)
- Hemoglobin A1c at least twice a year, but every three months if therapy has changed or glucose control is not at goal
- Flu shots

Additionally, the 2015 ADA guidelines recommend:
- Pneumococcal vaccination.
- Hepatitis B vaccine for unvaccinated adults who are 19–59 years of age.
- Weight loss for all overweight type 2 diabetic adults. How? By reducing energy intake (calories) while eating healthfully. "Weight-loss studies have used a variety of energy-restricted eating patterns, with no clear evidence that one eating pattern or optimal macronutrient distribution was ideal, suggesting that macronutrient proportions should be individualized."
- "Monitoring carbohydrate intake, whether by carbohydrate counting or experience-based estimation, remains a key strategy in achieving glycemic control."
- Limit alcohol to one (women) or two (men) drinks a day.
- "It is the position of the ADA that there is not a one-size-fits-all eating pattern for individuals with diabetes."
- "Individuals with type 1 diabetes should be offered intensive insulin therapy education

using the carbohydrate-counting meal planning approach, which has been shown to improve glycemic control. Consistent carbohydrate intake with respect to time and amount can result in improved glycemic control for individuals using fixed daily insulin doses."

- Foods containing sucrose (table sugar) should be minimized "...to avoid displacing nutrient-dense food choices."
- Diabetics and prediabetics should avoid sugar-sweetened beverages "...to reduce risk for weight gain and worsening of cardiometabolic risk profile."
- Monitoring carbohydrate intake is critical to achieving blood sugar control. The availability of insulin is also key.
- "A Mediterranean-style eating pattern, rich in monounsaturated fatty acids, may benefit glycemic control and cardiovascular disease risk factors and can therefore be recommended as an effective alternative to a lower-fat, higher-carbohydrate eating pattern."
- The ADA recommends an increase in foods containing long-chain omega-3 fatty acids (from fatty fish) and omega-3 linolenic acid (ALA).
- Fish consumption twice a week, particularly fatty fish (high omega-3 fatty acid), is recommended.
- Routine omega-3 fatty acid supplementation has not been shown to prevent or treat heart disease in diabetics.
- There is little evidence that blood sugars improve with routine supplementation with vitamin D, chromium, magnesium, or cinnamon or other herbs.
- The ideal amount of protein consumption for diabetics is unclear.

- Restriction of dietary protein is no longer routinely recommended in people with diabetic kidney disease (nephropathy with albuminuria). Instead, the focus is on control of blood pressure and blood sugar to prevent progression.
- During the initial diabetic exam, screen for peripheral arterial disease (poor circulation). Strongly consider calculation of the ankle-brachial index for those over 50 years of age; consider it for younger patients if they have risk factors for poor circulation.
- Those at risk for diabetes, including prediabetics, should aim for a) moderate weight loss if overweight (about seven percent of body weight), b) exercise: 150 minutes per week of moderate-intensity aerobic activity.
- "A variety of eating patterns have been shown to be effective in managing diabetes, including Mediterranean-style, Dietary Approaches to Stop Hypertension (DASH)-style, plant-based (vegan or vegetarian), lower-fat, and lower-carbohydrate patterns."

Clearly, some of my dietary recommendations you've read in this book conflict with ADA guidelines. The experts assembled by the ADA to compose guidelines were well-intentioned, intelligent, and hardworking. The guidelines are supported by hundreds of scientific journal references. I greatly appreciate the expert panel's work. We've simply reached some different conclusions. By the same token, I'm sure the expert panel didn't have unanimous agreement on all the final recommendations. I invite you to review the dietary guidelines yourself, discuss with your personal physician, then decide where you stand.

GENERAL TREATMENT GOALS

The ADA in 2015 suggests general therapeutic goals for adult non-pregnant diabetics:

- Blood pressure: under 140 mmHg systolic and under 90 mmHg diastolic
- LDL cholesterol: under 100 mg/dl (2.6 mmol/l). (In established cardiovascular disease: <70 mg/dl or 1.8 mmol/l.)
- HDL cholesterol: over 40 mg/dl (1.0 mmol/l) for men and over 50 mg/dl (1.3 mmol/l) for women
- Triglycerides: under 150 mg/dl (1.7 mmol/l)

Recommended blood sugar and hemoglobin A1c treatment goals were discussed in chapter 12.

IN CONCLUSION

Remember when you first found out you had diabetes or prediabetes? Maybe you knew just enough to be scared to death, with visions of amputations, endless needles, dialysis, and a life cut short.

You're moving in the right direction now!

This is an exciting time to have diabetes or prediabetes. We've come a long way since Dr. John Rollo's low-carb diet of 1797 (52) and Banting and Best's discovery of insulin in 1921 (53). As we learn more about underlying disease mechanisms, new therapies are being discovered every few years by unrelenting scientists. The pace of advancement is accelerating.

Diabetics today will not face the rates of amputation, blindness, kidney failure, and premature death seen too often in the past.

It can only get better.

###

REFERENCES

1. http://robbwolf.com/2011/10/17/type-1-diabetes-the-numbers-dont-lie/
2. http://www.dallasobserver.com/1995-07-06/news/neander-guy/
3. http://richthediabetic.com/paleo-is-helping-my-diabetes/
4. http://wholehealthsource.blogspot.com/2012/02/interview-with-dr-c-vicky-beer-paleo.html)
5. http://www.diabetes-warrior.net/about-me-and-diabetes/
6. http://paleolithicmd.com/2012/08/09/how-has-my-transition-to-paleo-changed-my-approach-to-treating-the-big-three-in-my-patients/
7. http://thecuriouscoconut.com/blog/my-journey-back-to-health
8. http://www.paleoinfused.com/?p=2454
9. http://www.paleoinfused.com/?p=2526
10. http://www.paleoinfused.com/?p=2425
11. http://paleoeater.blogspot.com/2008/11/paleo-diet-day-365-final-blog-entry.html
12. http://blog.joslin.org/2014/05/guest-blog-post-paleo-and-type-1-diabetes/
13. http://www.drkrunyan.com/About.html
14. http://www.everydayhealth.com/columns/type-two-and-you/how-reversed-prediabetes-discovered-new-passion-fitness-doctors-perspective/?xid=tw_everydayhealth_sf
15. http://thebloodsugarwhisperer.wordpress.com/2013/09/25/to-be-or-not-to-be-paleobetic/
16. http://robbwolf.com/2012/10/24/shades-paleo/
17. http://nycpastor.com/become-a-christian/

18. Mercader, Julio, et al. Mozambican grass seed consumption during the Middle Stone Age. *Science*, December 18, 2009.
19. http://advancedmediterranean.com/2012/02/22/are-saturated-fats-really-all-that-bad/
20. Konner, Melvin and Eaton, S. Boyd. Paleolithic nutrition: Twenty-five years later. *Nutrition in Clinical Practice*, 25 (2010): 594–602. doi: 10.1177/0884533610385702
21. Kuipers, R., et al (L. Cordain and S. Eaton are co-authors). Estimated macronutrient and fatty acid intakes from an East African Paleolithic diet. *British Journal of Nutrition*, (2010): 1–22 doi: 10.1017/S0007114510002679
22. Cordain, L., et al. Plant-animal subsistence ratios and macronutrient energy estimations in worldwide hunter-gatherer diets. *American Journal of Clinical Nutrition*, 71 (2000): 682–692.
23. http://thepaleodiet.com/the-paleo-diet-premise/
24. Blasbalg, T.L., et al. Changes in consumption of omega-3 and omega-6 fatty acids in the United States during the 20th century." *American Journal of Clinical Nutrition*, 93(2011): 950–962. doi:10.3945/ajcn.110.006643.
25. Figures are from an April 5, 2011, infographic at Civil Eats: http://www.civileats.com.
26. Kuipers, R.S., et al. A multidisciplinary reconstitution of Palaeolithic nutrition that holds promise for the prevention and treatment of diseases of civilization. *Nutrition Research Reviews*, 25(2012): 96–129.
27. Spreadbury, Ian. Comparison with ancestral diets suggests dense acellular carbohydrates promote an inflammatory microbiota, and may be the primary dietary cause of leptin resistance and obesity. *Diabetes, Metabolic Syndrome, and Obesity: Targets and Therapy* 5(2012): 175–189. doi: 10.2147/DMSO.S33473 http://www.ncbi.nlm.nih.gov/pmc/articles/PMC3402009/
28. Basu, S., Yoffe, P., Hills, N., Lustig, R.H. The relationship of sugar to population-level diabetes preva-

lence: An econometric analysis of repeated cross-sectional data. 8(2013) PLoS ONE: e57873. doi:10.1371/journal.pone.0057873.
29. http://care.diabetesjournals.org/content/early/2013/09/23/dc13-1397.abstract.html?papetoc
30. http://www.sorrentinodental.com/blog.html?entry=why-teeth-decay-i
31. http://www.npr.org/blogs/health/2013/02/24/172688806/ancient-chompers-were-healthier-than-ours
32. http://www.huffingtonpost.ca/mark-burhenne/paleo-diet-oral-health_b_4041350.html
33. Singh, G.M., et al. Mortality due to sugar-sweetened beverage consumption: A global, regional, and national comparative risk assessment. American Heart Association Epidemiology and Prevention/Nutrition, Physical Activity and Metabolism 2013 Scientific Sessions, Abstract EPI-13-A-879-AHA.
34. Mayo Clinic website, published October 16, 2012. http://www.mayoclinic.org/news2012-rst/7128.html
35. Eaton, S. Boyd, and Eaton, Stanley B. An evolutionary perspective on human physical activity: implications for health. *Comparative Biochemistry and Physiology: Part A Molecular and Integrative Physiology*, 136 (2003): 153–159.
36. Consider "Growing Stronger: Strength Training for Older Adults" http://www.cdc.gov/physicalactivity/downloads/growing_stronger.pdf
37. http://ren-ex.com/wp-content/uploads/2010/11/Exercise-vs-Recreation.pdf
38. O'Dea, Kerin. Marked improvement in carbohydrate and lipid metabolism in diabetic Australian Aborigines after temporary reversion to traditional lifestyle. *Diabetes*, 33 (1984): 596–603.
39. Lindeberg, S., Jönsson, T., Granfeldt, Y., Borgstrand, E., Soffman, J., Sjöström, K., & Ahrén, B. (2007). A Palaeolithic diet improves glucose tolerance more than a Mediterranean-like diet in individuals

with ischaemic heart disease. *Diabetologia*, 50 (2007): 1795–1807. doi 10.1007/s00125-007-0716-y

40. Österdahl, M; Kocturk, T; Koochek, A;Wändell, PE. Effects of a short-term intervention with a paleolithic diet in healthy volunteers. *European Journal of Clinical Nutrition*, 62 (2008): 682–685.

41. Jönsson, T., Granfeldt, Y., Ahrén, B., Branell, U., Pålsson, G., Hansson, A., Söderström, M., and Lindeberg, S. Beneficial effects of a Paleolithic diet on cardiovascular risk factors in type 2 diabetes: a randomized cross-over pilot study. *Cardiovascular Diabetology*, 8 (2009) doi: 10.1186/1475-2840-8-35

42. Frassetto, L.A., et al. Metabolic and physiologic improvements from consuming a paleolithic, hunter-gatherer type diet. *European Journal of Clinical Nutrition*, advance online publication, February 11, 2009. doi: 10.1038/ejcn.2009.4

43. Jönsson, Tommy, et al. A paleolithic diet is more satiating per calorie than a Mediterranean-like diet in individuals with ischemic heart disease. *Nutrition and Metabolism*, 2010, 7:85. doi: 10.1186/1743-7075-7-85

44. Ryberg, M., et al. A Palaeolithic-type diet causes strong tissue-specific effects on ectopic fat deposition in obese postmenopausal women. *Journal of Internal Medicine*, 274 (2013): 67–76. doi: 10.1111/joim.12048

45. Mellberg, C., et al (including M. Ryberg and T. Olsson). Long-term effects of a Palaeolithic-type diet in obese postmenopausal women: a 2-year randomized trial. *European Journal of Clinical Nutrition*, advance online publication January 29, 2014. doi: 10.1038/ejcn.2013.290

46. Boers, Inga, et al. Favorable effects of consuming a Palaeolithic-type diet on characteristics of the metabolic syndrome: a randomized controlled pilot-study. *Lipids in Health and Disease*. 2014 Oct 11; 13:160. doi: 10.1186/1476-511X-13-160.

47. http://paleodiabetic.com/2015/01/06/paleolithic-diet-improved-metabolic-syndrome-in-just-two-weeks/

48. http://balancedbites.com/practical-paleo-recipe-nutrition-facts

49. Pories, Walter and Dohm, G. Lynis. Diabetes: Have we got it all wrong? Hyperinsulinism as the culprit: surgery provides the evidence. *Diabetes Care*, 35 (2012): 2438–2442.

50. Taylor, Roy. Type 2 diabetes: Etiology and reversibility. *Diabetes Care*, 36 (2013): 1047-1055.

51.
https://www.youtube.com/watch?v=VjQkqFSdDOc

52.
http://dartmed.dartmouth.edu/winter08/html/diabetes_detectives.php

53. http://www.sciencebasedmedicine.org/lessons-from-the-history-of-insulin/

54. http://paleodiabetic.com/paleobetic-diet/

55. Masharani, U., et al. Metabolic and physiologic effects from consuming a hunter-gatherer (Paleolithic)-type diet in type 2 diabetes. *European Journal of Clinical Nutrition*, advance online publication April 1, 2015. doi: 10.1038/ejcn.2015.39

56. Johnston, Carol, et al. Examination of the anti-glycemic properties of vinegar in healthy adults. (Nine of the 40 study subjects had type 2 diabetes.) *Annals of Nutrition and Metabolism*, 56 (2010): 74-79.

SCIENTIFIC SUPPORT FOR A PALEO-STYLE DIABETIC DIET

Very few scientific studies look at the effects of Paleolithic eating on diabetics. The ones we have involve small numbers of patients and short-term follow-up. Here they are, as of May, 2015. More are in the pipeline. I've included a few research reports that involve non-diabetics because they tell us about physiological effects of the paleo diet that may help diabetics. This section is fairly technical and not written in a style for the general reading public. I'll refer to the studies by the first named author and the year published.

O'DEA 1984

This classic scientific article is often cited by those who favor a Paleolithic diet for diabetics. Researcher Kerin O'Dea wondered if Australian Aborigines would see improvement in their diabetes if they returned to their ancestral diet and lifestyle (38).

You need to know that urbanized Australian Aboriginal communities have a high prevalence of type 2 diabetes. O'Dea writes:

> The change from an urban to a traditional lifestyle involves several factors that directly affect insulin sensitivity: increased physical activity, reduced energy intake and weight loss, and changes in the overall dietary composition. All of these factors improve insulin sensitivity and should, therefore, be of benefit to the insulin-resistant diabetic.

Ten urban type 2 diabetic and four non-diabetic full-blood Aborigines agreed to revert to their traditional lifestyle as hunter-gatherers in an isolated region of Australia for seven weeks. Average age was 53. Half of them were moderate to heavy alcohol drinkers. Average diabetic weight was 82 kg (180 lb); non-diabetics averaged 77 kg (169 lb). There were equal numbers of men and women. None of the diabetics was on insulin, and only one was on an oral diabetic drug (a sulfonylurea).

The study was carried out at Pantijan, the traditional land of these Aborigines. It's a day-and-a-half drive in a four-wheel-drive vehicle from Derby. At least it was in 1984.

For seven weeks, the participants ate only what they hunted or collected. Diet composition was dependent on whether they were travelling to the homeland (1.5 weeks), at the coastal location (2 weeks), or inland on the river (3.5 weeks). Protein sources were mainly beef, kangaroo, fish, birds, crocodiles, and turtles. Carbohydrate content ranged from under 5% to 33%. Protein content varied from 50 to 80%. Fat was 13 to 40%. So, very high protein and low-carb. Carb sources were yams, honey, and figs. Yams were the predominant carb source. They also eat yabbies (shrimp or crayfish, or "crawdads" if you're from Oklahoma). Average energy intake was a very low 1,200 calories a day.

The author implies this was the traditional Aboriginal diet.

What did they eat back home in the city? The main dietary components were flour, sugar, rice, carbonated drinks, alcoholic drinks (beer and port), powdered milk, cheap fatty meat, potatoes, onions, and variable contributions of other fresh fruit and vegetables. O'Dea estimates a macronutrient breakdown of 50% carb, 40% fat, and 10% protein (similar to the Standard American Diet, then).

What did O'Dea find out? Everyone lost weight, a group average of 8 kg (18 lb) over the seven weeks.

Fasting blood sugars fell in the diabetics from 11.6 mmol/l to 6.6 mmol/l (209 to 119 mg/dl). After-meal blood sugars also fell dramatically.

Fasting insulin levels fell from 23 to 12 mU/l.

Fasting triglycerides fell drastically.

HDL cholesterol fell significantly, whereas LDL cholesterol tended to rise.

O'Dea wrote that, "Under the conditions of the study it is difficult to separate out effects of dietary composition, low energy intake, and weight loss."

She estimates that experimental activity levels were probably higher than in the urban setting, but not dramatically more so. (She was with the participants throughout the experiment.)

The main carbohydrate sources in this ancestral diet were yams, honey, and figs. Modern Australian honey is probably similar to the honey of 100,000 years ago. But what about yams and figs?

These folks had to have been eating twice as many calories, at least, back in their urban environment. O'Dea didn't comment on how well the participants tolerated calorie restriction. Did they complain? Did they eat to satiety? They had no access to food other than what they could hunt and gather. Was food in short supply? It's not documented. You'd think O'Dea would mention these issues if they were a problem.

This particular ancestral diet was extremely high in protein: 50–80% of calories. Eaton and Konner suggest that an average ancestral diet provides only 25–30% of total calories from protein. A typical modern high-protein diet derives about 30% of calories from protein, compared with 15% in the standard American diet. Protein helps combat hunger. But halving caloric intake for seven weeks is extreme. Don't believe me? Just try it. This degree of caloric restriction by itself would tend to lower blood sugar levels and body weight in most humans, regardless of macronutrient ratios and ethnicity.

I know nothing about Australian Aborigines as an ethnic and genetic group. Is their diabetes similar to European diabetes? Pima Indian diabetes? East Asian diabetes?

O'Dea never called the study diet Paleolithic, but it sounds like one. It was a modern hunter-gatherer diet eaten by rural, isolated Australian Aboriginal communities.

This calorie-restricted, very-high-protein, natural diet was very effective for weight loss and blood sugar control in this tiny, seven-week study on a specific ethnic population. Caloric restriction may have been the most effective component of the lifestyle change. Restriction of refined sugars and starches may have helped also.

This ancestral diet was beneficial for a few Australian Aborigines. Are the lessons widely applicable? Not yet. As they say, "further studies are needed."

It does jibe with plenty of other research that shows severe calorie restriction leads to weight loss and lower blood sugar levels.

LINDEBERG 2007

A Paleolithic diet lowered blood sugar levels better than a control diet in coronary heart disease patients with elevated blood sugars, according to Swedish researchers (39).

About half of all patients with coronary heart disease—arteries blocked with atherosclerosis—have abnormal blood sugar metabolism. Lindeberg and associates wondered if a Paleolithic diet would lead to improved blood sugar levels in heart patients, compared to healthy, Mediterranean-style, Western diet.

Investigators at the University of Lund enrolled 38 male heart patients—average age 61—and randomized them to either a paleo diet or a "consensus" (Mediterranean-like) diet to be followed for 12 weeks. Average weight was 94 kg (207 lb). Nine participants dropped out before completing the study, so results are based on 29 participants. All subjects had either prediabetes or type 2 diabetes (the majority) but none were taking medications to lower blood sugar. Baseline hemoglobin A1c's were around 4.8% (normal). Average fasting blood sugar was 125 mg/dl (6.9 mmol/l); average sugar two hours after 75 g of oral glucose was 160 mg/dl (8.9 mmol/l).

The paleo diet was based on lean meat, fish, fruits, leafy and cruciferous vegetables, root vegetables (potatoes limited to two or fewer medium-sized per day), eggs, and nuts (no grains, rice, dairy products, salt, or refined fats and sugar).

The Mediterranean-like diet focused on low-fat dairy, whole grains, vegetables, fruits, potatoes, fatty fish, oils and margarines rich in monounsaturated fatty acids and alpha-linolenic acid.

Both groups were allowed up to one glass of wine daily.

No effort was made to restrict total caloric intake with a goal of weight loss.

What did the researchers find? Absolute carbohydrate consumption was 43% lower in the paleo group (134 g versus 231 g), and 23% lower in terms of total calorie consumption (40% versus 52%). Glycemic load was 47% lower in the paleo group (65 versus 122), mostly reflecting lack of cereal grains.

The paleo group ate significantly more nuts, fruit, and vegetables. The Mediterranean group ate significantly more cereal grains, oil, margarine, and dairy products.

Glucose control improved by 26% in the paleo group compared to 7% in the consensus group. The improvement was statistically significant only in the paleo group. The researchers believe the improvement was independent of energy consumption, glycemic load, and dietary carb/protein/fat percentages.

High fruit consumption in the paleo group (493 g versus 252 g daily) didn't seem to impair glucose tolerance.

Hemoglobin A1c's didn't change or differ significantly between the groups.

Neither group showed a change in insulin sensitivity (by HOMA-IR method).

The authors' bottom line:

> In conclusion, we found marked improvement of glucose tolerance in ischemic heart disease patients with increased blood glucose or diabetes after advice to follow a Palaeolithic [sic] diet compared with a healthy Western diet. The larger improvement of glucose tolerance in the Palaeolithic group was independent of energy intake and macronutrient composition, which suggests that avoiding Western foods is more important than counting calories, fat, carbohydrate or protein. The study adds to the notion that healthy diets based on whole-grain cereals and low-fat dairy products are only the second

best choice in the prevention and treatment of type 2 diabetes.

This was a small study; I consider it a promising pilot. Results apply to men only, and perhaps only to Swedish men. I have no reason to think they wouldn't apply to women, too. Who knows about other ethnic groups?

The Mediterranean-style consensus diet here included low-fat dairy and margarine, items I don't associate with the traditional healthy Mediterranean diet.

The higher fruit consumption of the paleo group didn't adversely affect glucose control, which is surprising. Fruit is supposed to raise blood sugar. At 493 grams a day, men in the paleo group ate almost seven times the average fruit intake of Swedish men in the general population (75 g/day). Perhaps lack of adverse effect on glucose control here reflects that these diabetics and prediabetics were in fact mild cases early in the course of the condition. They still had a significant degree of pancreas beta cell function, so they could handle the sugar in the fruit. A type 2 diabetic late in the course of the disease, taking two, three, or more diabetes drugs, may have had worse blood sugar control than these study participants

Present day paleo and low-carb diet advocates share some overlap, mostly because of carbohydrate restriction—at least to some degree—by paleo dieters. Both groups favor natural, relatively unprocessed foods. Note that the average American eats 250–300 g of carbohydrates a day. Total carb intake in the paleo group was only yp134 g (40% of calories) versus 231 g (55% of calories) in the Mediterranean-style diet. Other versions of the paleo diet will yield different numbers, as will individual choices for various fruits and vegetables. Forty percent of total energy consumption from carbs barely qualifies as low-carb.

Study participants were mild, diet-controlled diabetics or prediabetics, not representative of the overall diabetic population, most of whom take drugs for it and have much higher hemoglobin A1c's.

The paleo diet shows promise as a treatment or preventative for prediabetes and type 2 diabetes. Only time will tell if it's better long-term—in terms of lower mortality and fewer diabetic complications—than a low-carb Mediterranean diet or other low-carb diets.

OSTERDAHL 2008

Swedish investigators at Karolinska Institutet found diminished weight, body mass index, blood pressure, and waist circumference in 14 healthy medical students eating a paleo diet for three weeks (40). This is one of the seminal scientific clinical studies of the paleo diet in modern Europeans.

Their version of the paleo diet:
- Allowed ad lib: All fresh or frozen fruits, berries and vegetables except legumes, canned tomatoes without additives, fresh or frozen unsalted fish and seafood, fresh or frozen unsalted lean meats and minced meat, unsalted nuts (except peanuts, a legume), fresh squeezed lemon or lime juice (as dressing), flaxseed or rapeseed oil (as dressing), coffee and tea (without sugar, milk, honey, or cream), all salt-free spices.
- Allowed but with major restrictions: dried fruit, salted seafood, fat meat, potatoes (two medium-sized per day), honey, cured meats
- Prohibited: all milk and dairy products, all grain products (including corn and rice), all legumes, canned food except tomatoes, candy, ice cream, soft drinks, juices, syrups, alcohol, sugar, and salt

What did the researchers find?

- Average weight dropped from 65.2 kg (144 lb) to 62.9 (139 lb)
- Average body mass index fell from 22.2 to 21.4
- Average waist circumference decreased from 74.3 cm (29.25 inches) to 72.6 cm (28.58 inches)
- Average systolic blood pressure fell from 110 to 104 mmHg
- plasminogen activator inhibitor-1 decreased from 5.0 kIE/l to 2.8 kIE/l

All of these changes were statistically significant. The researchers looked at a number of other blood tests and didn't find any significant differences.

Five men and nine women completed the study. Of the 20 who originally signed up, one couldn't fulfill the diet, three became ill (no details), two failed to show up.

So what? That's a remarkable weight loss over just three weeks for slender people eating ad lib.

The study authors concluded that these paleo diet-induced changes could reduce risk for cardiovascular disease.

What does this study have to do with diabetes? Type 2 diabetics and prediabetics are often overweight, at increased risk for heart disease, and need to lower their blood pressure. Type 1s are at increased risk of heart disease. The paleo diet may help move things in the right direction.

JONSSON 2009

Compared to a standard diabetic diet, a Paleolithic diet improved cardiovascular risk factors in type 2 diabetics, according to investigators at Lund University in Sweden (41).

Researchers compared the effects of a paleo and a modern diabetic diet in 13 type 2 diabetic adults (10 men) with average hemoglobin A1c's of 6.6% (under fairly good control, then). Most were on diabetic pills; none were on insulin. So this was a small, exploratory, pilot study. Each of the diabetics followed both diets for three months.

How did the diets differ? Compared to the diabetic diet, the paleo diet was mainly lower in cereals and dairy products, higher in fruits and vegetables, meat, and eggs. The paleo diet was lower in carbohydrates, glycemic load, and glycemic index. Paleo vegetables were primarily leafy and cruciferous. Cruciferous vegetables include broccoli, brussels sprouts, cauliflower, and cabbage. Root vegetables were allowed; up to 1 medium potato daily. The paleo diet also featured lean meats, fish, eggs, and nuts, while forbidding refined fats, sugars, and beans. Up to one glass of wine daily was allowed.

See the actual report for details of the standard diabetic diet, which seems to me to be similar to the diabetic diet recommended by most U.S. dietitians.

What did the researchers find? Compared to the diabetic diet, the paleo diet yielded lower hemoglobin A1c's (0.4% lower), lower trigylcerides, lower diastolic blood pressure, lower weight, lower body mass index, lower waist circumference, lower total energy (caloric) intake, and higher HDL cholesterol (the good cholesterol). Glucose tolerance was the same for both diets. Fasting blood sugars tended to decrease more on the Paleo diet, but did not reach statistical significance (p=0.08, which is very close to significant).

So what? The greater improvement in multiple cardiovascular risk factors seen here suggests that the paleo diet has potential to reduce the higher cardiovascular disease rates we see in diabetics. This is just a pilot study. Larger studies—more participants—are needed for confirmation. Ultimately, we need data on hard clinical endpoints such as heart attacks, strokes, and death.

These diabetics had their blood sugars under fairly good control at baseline. I wouldn't be surprised if diabetics under poor control—hemoglobin A1c of 9%, for example—would see even greater improvements in risk factors as well as glucose levels while eating paleo-style.

This study suggests the paleo diet may help with weight loss.

There are so few women in this study as to be almost meaningless. Results of this study may or may not apply to non-Swedes.

FRASSETTO 2009

A Paleolithic diet improved metabolic status with respect to cardiovascular and carbohydrate physiology, according to investigators at the University of California San Francisco (42).

This was a small, preliminary study: only nine participants (six male, three female, all healthy (non-diabetic), average age 38, average BMI 28 (overweight), sedentary, mixed Black/Caucasian/Asian).

Baseline diet characteristics were determined by dietitians, then all participants were placed on a paleo diet, starting with a 7-day ramp-up (increasing fiber and potassium gradually), then a 10-day paleo diet.

The paleo diet: meat, fish, poultry, eggs, fruits, vegetables, tree nuts, canola oil, mayonnaise, and honey. No dairy, legumes, cereals, grains, potatoes. Alcohol wasn't mentioned ever. Caloric intake was adjusted to avoid weight change during the study, and participants were told to remain sedentary. They ate one meal daily at the research center and were sent home with the other meals and snacks pre-packed.

Compared with baseline diets, the paleo diet reduced salt consumption by half while doubling potassium and magnesium intake. Baseline diet macronutrient calories were 17% from protein, 44% carbohydrate, 38% fat. Paleo diet macronutrients were 30% protein, 38% carb, 32% fat. Fiber content wasn't reported.

What did the researchers find? Here are the specific changes linked to the paleo diet, all statistically significant unless otherwise noted:

- total cholesterol decreased by 16%
- LDL cholesterol ("bad cholesterol") decreased by 22% (no change in HDL)
- triglycerides decreased by 35%
- strong trend toward reduced fasting insulin (P=0.07), but not quite statistically significant
- average diastolic blood pressure down by 3 mmHg (no change in systolic pressure)
- improved insulin sensitivity and reduced insulin resistance; i.e., improved glucose tolerance

I'm guessing there were no adverse effects.

This study sounds like fun, easy, basic science: "Hey, let's do this and see what happens!"

Canola oil is considered one of the healthy oils by folks like Walter Willett at Harvard. It sounds more appealing than rapeseed, from whence it comes.

I agree with the investigators that this tiny preliminary study is promising; the paleo diet has potential benefits for prevention and treatment for metabolic syndrome, diabetes, and cardiovascular disease such as heart attack and stroke.

JONSSON 2010

Swedish researchers report that a Paleolithic diet was more satiating than a Mediterranean-style diet, when compared on a calorie-for-calorie basis in heart patients (43). Both groups of study subjects reported equal degrees of satiety, but the paleo dieters ended up eating 24% fewer calories over the 12-week study.

Participants had mild diabetes or prediabetes. The diabetics had mild disease controlled by diet alone: average hemoglobin A1c of all participants was 4.7 (normal). Average starting weight of these 29 ischemic heart patients was 93 kg (205 lb). Each intervention group had only 13 or 14 patients.

The paleo dieters were advised to increase their intake of lean meat, fish, vegetables and fruit, and to avoid all dairy products, cereals (including rice), beans, bakery products, sugar, beer, and soft drinks. The following items were acceptable but limited: nuts (walnuts preferred), eggs (up to one per day), potatoes (two or fewer medium-sized per day), olive or rapeseed oil (one or fewer tablespoons per day). No advice was given with regard to proportions of food categories (e.g. plant versus animal foods).

Both the paleo dieters and Mediterranean dieters could eat as much as they wanted.

The main differences in the diets were that the paleo dieters had much lower consumption of cereals (grains) and dairy products, and more fruit and nuts. The paleos derived 40% of total calories from carbohydrate compared to 52% among the Mediterraneans.

Even though it wasn't a weight-loss study, both groups lost weight. The paleo dieters lost a bit more than the Mediterraneans: 5 kg vs 3.8 kg (11 lb vs 8.4 lb). That's fantastic weight loss for people not even trying.

As I slogged through the research report, I had to keep reminding myself that this is a very small, pilot study. So I'll not bore you with all the details.

Bottom line? This study suggests that the paleo diet may be particularly helpful for weight loss in heart patients with prediabetes and mild type 2 diabetes. No one knows how results would compare a year or two after starting the diet. The typical weight-loss pattern is to start gaining the weight back at six months, with return to baseline at one or two years out.

Many diabetics, particularly if they have type 2, are overweight or obese. The study at hand suggests that the paleo diet my help with weight loss, which in turn may help control diabetes, improve cardiovascular disease risk factors, and reduce the need for diabetes drugs. We have 12 classes of drugs for treating type 2 diabetes, and we don't know the long-term adverse effects of most of them.

Greek investigators found a link between the Mediterranean diet and better clinical outcomes in known ischemic heart disease patients. On the other hand, researchers at the Heart Institute of Spokane found the Mediterranean diet equivalent to a low-fat diet in heart patients, again in terms of clinical outcomes. U.S. investigators in 2007 found a positive link between the Mediterranean diet and lower rates of death from cardiovascular disease and cancer.

We don't yet have these kinds of studies looking at the potential benefits of the paleo diet. I'm talking about hard clinical endpoints such as heart attacks, heart failure, cardiac deaths, and overall deaths. The paleo diet definitely shows some promise.

I also note the Swedish investigators didn't point out that weight loss in overweight heart patients may be detrimental. This is the "obesity paradox."

RYBERG 2013

This study (44) didn't involve diabetics, but gives us some clues that the paleo diet may help with management of overweight postmenopausal women who have or are at risk for prediabetes, type 2 diabetes, high blood pressure, and heart disease.

After menopause, body fat in women tends to accumulate more centrally (in the abdomen) than peripherally. This is reflected in a higher incidence of fatty liver disease, type 2 diabetes, and cardiovascular disease. A multinational group of researchers wondered if a modified paleo-style diet would have metabolic effects on healthy overweight and obese (BMI 28–35) postmenopausal women in Sweden, with particular attention to fat levels in liver and muscle.

Curiously, they researchers never give the age range of the 10 study participants. Were they closer to 52 or 82?

The five-week intervention diet seems to have been mostly prepared and provided by the investigators, but they allowed for home cooking by providing menus, recipes, and a food list. No limit on consumption. The goal was to obtain 30% of calories from protein, 40% from fat (mostly unsaturated), and 30% from carbohydrate "...together with 40 g nuts (walnuts and sweet almonds) on a daily basis...."

The diet included lean meat, fish, fruit, vegetables (including root vegetables), eggs and nuts. The following were excluded: dairy products, cereals, beans, refined fats and sugar, added salt, bakery products, and soft drinks.

"They were also advised to use only rapeseed [i.e., canola] or olive oil in food preparation."

A diet like this should reduce average saturated fat consumption, which was a stated goal, while substituting monounsaturated and polyunsaturated fat for saturated.

These women were sedentary before and during the intervention.

What did the researchers find? The ladies indeed made some major changes in their diet. Total calories consumed fell by 22% (2,400 to 1,900 calories). The average weight of participants dropped from 190 lb (86.4 kg) to 180 lb (81.8 kg).

Carbohydrates consumption as a percentage of total calories fell from 49% to 25%. Total carb grams dropped from 281 to 118, with fiber grams unchanged. To replace some of the carbs, the women increased their protein and fat calorie percentages by about a third. The authors don't make it clear whether the total carb grams included total fiber grams. "Before" and "after" fiber grams were 25 and 27, respectively.

In other words, "...the ratio between energy intake from the macronutrients protein, total fat and carbohydrates expressed as E% [calorie percentages] changed significantly from 16:33:50 at baseline to 28:44:25 after five weeks." Total daily fat grams didn't change, but the contribution of saturated fat grams fell.

A 10-point drop in systolic blood pressure over the five weeks didn't quite reach statistical significance (p=0.057), but the 9% drop in diastolic pressure did.

"Fasting serum levels of glucose, leptin, cholesterol, triglycerides, HDL, LDL, ApoB and apolipoprotein A1 (ApoA1) and percentage HDL also decreased significantly."

Fat (or lipid) content of the liver dropped by half. It was measured by magnetic resonance spectroscopy. Peripheral muscle fat content didn't change, measured in the soleus and tibialis anterior muscles of the leg.

"Urinary C-peptide excretion and HOMA indices [HOMA1-IR formula] decreased significantly, whereas whole-body insulin sensitivity, measured using the hyperinsulinaemic euglycaemic clamp technique, was not significantly changed."

I have lots of comments.

The intervention diet was a reasonable version of the Paleolithic diet, with one exception: canola oil has fallen out of favor. It's highly processed and didn't exist even a hundred years ago. From what I've seen from Eaton, Konner, and Cordain, I think they'd agree.

My fantasy about extra virgin olive oil is that it simply oozes out of the olives when pressure is applied. So easy a caveman could do it.

Eaton and Konner have argued that our ancestral diet would have had at least two or three times the fiber as was provided by this diet. But that would have been at a total daily calorie consumption level of at least 3,000 or 3,500 back in the day. So this diet isn't so far off.

The 10 lb (4.6 kg) weight loss over five weeks is impressive for an eat-all-you-want diet. Calorie intake dropped spontaneously by 500/day, assuming the numbers are accurate. The satiation from higher protein consumption may explain that. The authors admit that the women lost more weight than would be predicted by the energy balance equation (i.e., a pound of fat = 3,500 calories). They wonder about overestimations of food intake, thermogenic effects of protein versus other macronutrients, and loss of glycogen (and associated body water). You can't argue with those scales, though.

While serum C-peptide didn't fall, urinary levels did. My sense from reviewing other literature is that 24-hr urine levels of C-peptide are more accurate indicators of insulin production, compared to a single fasting C-peptide level. The authors interpret this as increased insulin sensitivity in the liver in combination with decreased insulin secretion by the pancreas. Fasting serum insulin levels fell from 8.35 to 6.75 mIU/l (p<0.05). Overall, these would tend to be beneficial changes for prediabetics and diabetics.

Regarding the non-significant change in overall insulin sensitivity as judged by hyperinsulinemic euglycemic clamp technique, remember that insulin sensitivity of the liver may be different from sensitivity in peripheral tissues such as muscle. These investigators think that liver insulin sensitivity was clearly improved with their diet.

Blood lipid changes were in the right direction in terms of cardiovascular disease risk, except for the drops in HDL (from 1.35 to 1.17 mmol/l) and ApoA1.

This study may or may not apply to men. Also note the small sample size. Will these results be reproducible in a larger population? In different ethnicities?

I like the reduction in blood pressure. That could help you avoid the risk, expense, and hassle of drug therapy.

I like the drop in fasting blood sugar from 96 to 90 mg/dl (5.35 to 5 mmol/l). It's modest, but statistically significant. Was it caused by the weight loss, reduced total carb consumption, paucity of sugar and refined starches, lower total calories, higher consumption of protein and mono- and polyunsaturated fats, or a combination of factors? As with most nutritional studies, there's a lot going on here. A small fasting blood sugar drop like this wouldn't matter to most type 2 diabetics, but could diabetics see an even greater reduction than these non-diabetics? Only one way to tell: do the study.

I can well imagine this diet curing some cases of metabolic syndrome, prediabetes, mild type 2 diabetes, and fatty liver disease.

Most type 2 diabetics (and prediabetics, for that matter) are overweight or obese. If a diet like this helps them lose weight, it could improve blood sugar levels. Nearly all authorities recommend that overweight and obese diabetics and prediabetics get their weight down to normal. (I admit that weight loss and improved blood sugar levels are not always in sync.) Weight loss by any standard method tends to improve insulin sensitivity.

Furthermore, the elevated fasting blood sugars that characterize so many cases of diabetes and prediabetes are usually linked to, if not caused by, insulin resistance in the liver. According to these investigators, the diet at hand improves insulin sensitivity in the liver, and even lowers fasting blood sugars in non-diabetic older women.

This modified Paleolithic-style diet doesn't include table sugar or refined grain starches. That would help control blood sugar levels in both type 1 and type 2 diabetics and prediabetics. The authors didn't say so, but this must be a relatively low-glycemic-index diet.

The investigators don't mention ramifications of their diet for folks with diabetes. Their focus is on ectopic fat accumulation (in liver and muscle) and its linkage with insulin resistance and cardiovascular disease. They've put together a promising program to try on diabetics or prediabetics. They just need the will and funding to get it done.

I agree with the authors that the lower calorie consumption, rather than the paleo diet per se, may have caused or contributed to the reduction in liver fat.

The investigators wonder if a Paleolithic-style diet like this would be beneficial over the long-term in patients with non-alcoholic fatty liver disease (NALFD) and associated metabolic disturbance (e.g., impaired insulin sensitivity in the liver). NAFLD tends to predict the development of diabetes and cardiovascular disease. If we can prevent or reverse fatty liver, we may prevent or reverse type 2 diabetes and cardiovascular disease, to an extent. You'll be waiting many years for those clinical study results. But you have to decide what to eat today.

A significant number of American women (20%?) need to lose weight, lower their blood pressures, lower their blood sugars, and decrease their liver fat. This Ryberg Paleolithic-style diet would probably do it.

A very-low-carb diet is another way to reduce liver fat, and it's more effective than simple calorie restriction.

MELLBERG 2014

Swedish researchers compared a Paleolithic-type diet against a lower-fat, higher-carb diet so often recommend in Nordic countries and in the U.S. (45). The investigators were interested in weight loss, cardiometabolic risk factors, and overall body composition. Test subjects were obese but otherwise healthy older women without diabetes. The study lasted two years. Dieters could eat as much as they wanted.

They found that the paleo-style dieters lost more weight, lost more abdominal fat, and lowered their trigyceride levels.

I don't know what the researchers told the women to get them interested. Weight loss versus healthier diet versus ? This could have influenced the type of women who signed up, and their degree of commitment.

A newspaper ad got the attention of 210 women in Sweden; 70 met the inclusion criteria, which included a body mass index 27 or higher and generally good health. Average age was 60. Average BMI was 33. Average weight was 87 kg (192 lb). Average waist circumference was 105 cm (41 inches). The women were randomized into one of two diet groups (N=35 in each): paleolithic-type diet (PD) or Nordic Nutrition Recommendations diet (NNR). There were no limits on total caloric consumption. (Were the women told to "work on weight loss"? I have no idea.)

We don't know the ethnicity of these women.

Here's their version of the paleo diet:
- 30% of energy (calories) from protein
- 40% of energy from fat
- 30% of energy from carbohydrate
- high intake of mono- and polyunsaturated fatty acids
- based on lean meat, fish, eggs, vegetables, fruits, berries, and nuts
- additional fat sources were avocado and oils (rapeseed [canola] and olive) used in dressings and food preparation
- cereals (grains), dairy products, added salt and refined fats and sugar were excluded
- no mention of legumes, potatoes, or tubers

The NNR diet:
- 15% of energy from protein
- 25–30% of energy from fat
- 55–60% of energy from carbohydrate
- emphasis on high-fiber products and low-fat dairy products

Over the 24 months of the study, each cohort had 12 group meetings with a dietitian for education and support, including "dietary effects on health, behavioral changes and group discussion."

Various blood tests and body measurements were made at baseline and periodically. Body measurements were made every six months. Body composition was measured by dual energy x-ray absorptiometry. Diet intake was measured by self-reported periodic four-day food records.

What did the researchers find? The paleo-style dieters lost more weight, lost more abdominal fat, and lowered their triglyceride levels. When measured six months into the study, the paleo dieters had lost 6.5 kg (14 lb) of body fat compared to 2.6 (6 lb) kg in the other group.

Measured at two years out, the paleo dieters had lost 4.6 kg (10 lb) of body fat compared to 2.9 kg (6 lb) in the other group, but this difference wasn't statistically significant.

The greatest weight loss was clocked at 12 months: Paleo dieters were down 8.7 (19 lb) kg compared to 4.4 kg (10 lb) in the other group.

Thirty percent of participants (21) eventually dropped out by the end of the study and were lost to follow-up, leaving 27 in the PD group and 22 in the NNR cohort.

Food record analysis indicated the PD group indeed reduced their carb intake while increasing protein and fat over baseline. Baseline macronutrient energy percentages were about the same for both groups: 17% protein, 45% carb, 34% (I guess the percentages don't add to 100 because of alcohol, which was not mentioned at all in the article.) Two years out, the PD group's energy sources were 22% protein, 34% carb, 40% fat. For the NNR group, the energy sources at two years were 17% protein, 43% carb, and 34% fat. As usual, dietary compliance was better at six months compared to 24 months. The PD group failed to reach target amounts of protein energy (30%) at six and 24 months; the NNR group didn't reach their goal of carbohydrate energy (55–60%). The PD group ate more mono- and poly unsaturated fatty acids than the NNRs.

In contrast to the food record estimates of protein intake, the urine tests for protein indicated poor adherence to the recommended protein consumption in the PD group (30% of energy). Both groups ate the same amount of protein by this metric. (This is an issue mostly ignored by authors, who don't say which method is usually more accurate.)

"Both groups had statistically significant weight loss during the whole study, with significantly greater weight loos in the PD group at all follow up time points except at 24 months." Largest weight loss was measured at 12 month: 8.7 kg (19 lb) in the PD group versus 4.4 kg (10 lb) in the NNRs.

The PD group lost 6.5 kg (14 lb) of body fat by six months but the loss was only 4.6 kg (10 lb) measured at 24 months. Corresponding numbers for the NNR group were 2.6 and 2.9 kg (about 6 lb). So both groups decreased their total fat mass to a significant degree. The difference between the groups was significant (P<0.001) only at six months. The greatest weight loss was clocked at 12 months: PD dieters were down 8.7 kg (19 lb) compared to 4.4 kg (10 lb) in the NNRs. Both groups saw a significant decrease in waist circumference during the whole study, with a more pronounce decrease in the PD group at six months: 11 versus 6 cm (4.3 versus 2.4 inches).

Fasting blood sugars, fasting insulin levels, and tissue plasminogen activator activity didn't change.

259

Both groups had improvements in blood pressure, heart rate, C-reactive protein, LDL cholesterol, PAI-1 activity, and total cholesterol. The PD group saw a greater drop in triglycerides (by 19% at two years, but levels were normal to start with at 108 mg/dl or 1.22 mmol/l).

Reported daily energy intake fell over time for both groups, without statistically significant differences between them.

As measured at six months, the paleo dieters lost 10% of their initial body weight, compared to 5% in the NNR group. That's worth something to many folks. However, the researchers didn't find much, if any, difference in the groups in terms of cardiometabolic risk factors. They wonder if that reflects the baseline healthiness of these women. Would a sicker study population show more improvement on one of the diets?

I'm surprised the NNR group lost any weight at all. In my experience it's hard for most folks to lose weight and keep it off while eating as much as they want, unless they're eating very-low-carb. We've seen short-term weight loss with ad libitum paleo diets before. I bet the women signing up for this study were highly motivated to change.

Legumes and potatoes are a debatable part of the paleo diet. Most versions exclude legumes. We don't know if these women ate legumes and potatoes. Other than this oversight, the experimental paleo diet is reasonable.

The authors noted that the paleo diet group failed to reach their protein intake goal (30% of total calories), and suggested reasons "such as protein-rich foods being more expensive, social influences on women's food choices or a lower food preference for protein-rich food among women."

The results of this study may or may not apply to other population subgroups and non-Swedes.

The authors write:

> In conclusion, a Palaeolithic-type [sic] diet during two years with ad libitum intake of macronutrients, including an increased intake of polyunsaturated fatty acids and monounsaturated fatty acids reduces fat mass and abdominal obesity with significantly better long-term effect on triglyceride levels vs an NNR diet. Adherence to the prescribed protein intake was poor in the PD group suggesting that other components of the PD diet are of greater importance.

Does this study have anything to do with diabetes? Not directly. But it suggests that if an overweight diabetic needs to lose excess body fat without strict calorie control, a lower-carb paleo-style diet may be more effective than the usual recommended low-fat, higher-carb diet. I would have liked to have seen lower fasting blood sugar and insulin levels in the paleo dieters, but wishing doesn't make it so.

BOERS 2014

A Paleolithic-type diet over just two weeks improved several diabetes and heart disease risk factors in obese folks with metabolic syndrome, according to Netherlands-based researchers (46).

The investigators wondered if the paleo diet, independent of weight loss, would alter characteristics of the metabolic syndrome.

"Metabolic syndrome" may be a new term for you. It's a collection of clinical features that are associated with increased future risk of type 2 diabetes and atherosclerotic complications such as heart attack and stroke. One of the metabolic syndrome criteria is elevated fasting blood sugar. One in six Americans has metabolic syndrome, including almost one in four adults. The most common definition of metabolic syndrome (and there are others) is the presence of at least three of the following characteristics:

- high blood pressure (130/85 or higher, or using a high blood pressure medication)
- low HDL cholesterol: under 40 mg/dl (1.03 mmol/l) in a man, under 50 mg/dl (1.28 mmol/l) in a women (or either sex taking a cholesterol-lowering drug)
- triglycerides over 150 mg/dl (1.70 mmol/l) (or taking a triglyceride-lowering drug)
- abdominal fat: waist circumference 40 inches (102 cm) or greater in a man, 35 inches (88 cm) or greater in a woman
- fasting blood glucose over 100 mg/dl (5.55 mmol/l)

These five criteria were identical to the ones used in the study at hand. But the study participants were required to have only two of the five, not three, for unclear reasons.

Average age of the 34 study participants was 53 and they were generally healthy. None had diabetes, cardiovascular disease, or systolic pressure over 180 mmHg. Mean body mass index was 32 (obese). Only 9 of the 34 subjects were men. Subjects were randomized to either a Paleolithic-type diet (n=18) or a "healthy reference diet based on the guidelines of the Dutch Health Council" (n=14). Efforts were made to keep body weight stable during the two-week study. Participants were nearly all Caucasian.

All meals were home-delivered free of charge by a catering service.

The Paleolithic-type diet "...was based on lean meat, fish, fruit, leafy and cruciferous vegetables, root vegetables, eggs and nuts. Dairy products, cereal grains, legumes, refined fats, extra salt and sugar were not part of it." (I like their version of the paleo diet.) Protein supplied 24% of calories while carbohydrate was 32% and fat 41%.

You can consult the full text of the published article for details of the Dutch Health Council diet. Calories were 17% from protein, 50% from carbohydrate, and 29% from fat. Alcohol isn't mentioned at all.

Despite randomization, the paleo diet group had more metabolic syndrome characteristics than the reference diet group. For instance, 78% of the paleo group had elevated fasting glucose compared to 44% of the reference group. And 67% of the paleo group had low HDL cholesterol compared to just 13% of the reference group. These glucose and HDL differences between groups were statistically significant. 39% of the paleo had high triglycerides compared to 19% of the others. Furthermore, the paleo's average body weight was 98 kg (216 lb) compared to 86 kg (189 lb) in the others. The paleo group had 3.7 characteristics of the metabolic syndrome versus 2.7 in the other cohort.

Overall, I'm not very pleased with this study. My biggest problems are 1) an unfortunate randomization process that created dissimilar experimental groups, 2) the use of two diet protocols, 3) some of the study participants didn't even have metabolic syndrome, and 4) as is typical for paleo diet studies, not many experimental subjects were involved. Analyzing this study was very frustrating and time-consuming for me. For my full analysis, see my Paleo Diabetic blog (47). I'll simplify things here.

The best way to look at this study is to consider it simply a paleo diet trial involving 18 subjects who had metabolic syndrome. If I'm interpreting Table 5 correctly, and I think I am, these are the statistically significant changes within the group after two weeks of the paleo diet:

- abdominal circumference decreased by 3.1 cm
- systolic and diastolic blood pressures dropped by 8.5 and 8, respectively
- fasting glucose dropped by 0.4 mmol/l (7 mg/dl)
- fasting insulin fell
- HOMA-IR decreased (less insulin resistance)
- total cholesterol decreased from 220 to 193 mg/dl (5.7 to 5.0 mmol/l)
- LDL-cholesterol decreased from 135 to 124 mg/dl (3.5 to 3.2 mmol/l)
- triglycerides decreased from 168 to 89 mg/dl (1.9 to 1.0 mmol/l)
- HDL-cholesterol was unchanged

The fall in AUC (area under the curve) for insulin approached but didn't reach statistical significance (p=0.08).

Body weight fell from 98 kg to 95.3 kg (216 to 210 lb) but I found no p value. That's an amazing weight loss since the investigators were taking measures to avoid weight loss.

All of these changes (except the lack of change in HDL-cholesterol) would tend to promote health in someone with metabolic syndrome, prediabetes, or overweight type 2 diabetes.

Masharani 2015

A three-week Paleolithic-style diet improved blood sugars and lipids in obese type 2 diabetics, according to researchers at the University of California—San Francisco (55). I believe Lynda Frassetto was the leader of the team.

To understand the impact of this study, you need to know about a blood test called fructosamine, which reflects blood sugar levels over the preceding 2–3 weeks. You may already be familiar with a blood test called hemoglobin A1c: it tells us about blood sugars over the preceding three months. Blood glucose binds to proteins in our blood in a process called glycation. The higher the blood glucose, the more bonding. Glucose bound to hemoglobin molecules is measured in hemoglobin A1c (HgbA1c). Glucose bound to plasma proteins—predominantly albumin—is measured as fructosamine. It probably has nothing to do with fructose. Fructosamine is a generic name for plasma ketoamines.

If you're doing a diabetic diet study over 2–3 weeks, like the report at hand, changes in glucose control will mostly be detected in fructosamine rather than HgbA1c levels.

Twenty-five obese diabetics in the San Francisco Bay area were randomly assigned to either a paleo-style diet or one based on American Diabetes Association (ADA) guidelines. They followed the diets for three weeks, with various measurements taken before and after intervention.

Participants were aged 50–69. Sex of the study subjects was not specified. Average body mass index was 34. Over half (63%) were White/European American; there were three each of Asian, African American, and Hispanic ethnicity. They had normal blood pressures and diabetes was well controlled, with hemoglobin A1c's around 7% and fructosamine levels close to normal. Four subjects were on no diabetes medications, 14 were taking metformin alone, five were on metformin and a sulfonylurea, one was on long-acting insulin and a sulfonylurea. No drug dosages were changed during the study.

Both intervention diets were designed for weight maintenance, i.e., avoidance of weight loss or gain. If participants lost weight, they were instructed to eat more. All food was prepared and provided for the par-

265

ticipants. Three meals and three snacks were provided for daily consumption.

Fourteen subjects completed the paleo diet intervention. They ate lean meats, fruits, vegetables, tree nuts, poultry, eggs, canola oil, mayonnaise, and honey. No added salt. No cereal grains, dairy, legumes, or potatoes. Calorie percentages from protein, fat, and carbohydrate were 18%, 27%, and 58%, respectively. Compared to the ADA diet, the paleo diet was significantly lower in saturated fat, calcium, and sodium (under half as much), while higher in potassium (twice as much). These dieters eased into the full paleo diet over the first week, allowing bodies to adjust to higher fiber and potassium consumption. The paleo diet had about 40 grams of fiber, over twice as much as the ADA diet.

Ten subjects completed the ADA diet, which included moderate salt, low-fat dairy, whole grains, rice, bread, legumes, and pasta. Calorie percentages from protein, fat, and carbohydrate were 20%, 29%, and 54%, respectively (very similar to the paleo diet). I don't have any additional description for you. I assume it included meat, poultry, eggs, and fruit.

Diet compliance was confirmed via urine measurements of sodium, potassium, pH, and calcium.

What did the researchers find?

Both groups on average lost about 2 kg (4–5 lb).

Compared to their baseline values, the paleo group saw reductions in total cholesterol, HDL cholesterol, LDL cholesterol, HgbA1c (down 0.3% absolute reduction), and fructosamine. Fructosamine fell from 294 to 260 micromole/L. (The normal non-diabetic range for fructosamine is 190-270 micromole/L.)

Compared to their baseline values, the ADA diet group saw reductions in HDL cholesterol and HgbA1c (down

0.2% absolute reduction) but no change in fructosa-mine, total cholesterol, and LDL cholesterol.

Comparing the groups to each other, the difference in fructosamine change was right on the cusp of statisti-cal significance at p = 0.06.

Within each group, insulin resistance trended down, but didn't reach statistical significance. However, when they looked at the folks who were the most insulin re-sistant, only the paleo dieters improved their re-sistance. By the way, insulin resistance was measure via euglycemic hyperinsulinemic clamp instead of the short-cut HOMA-IR method.

Blood pressures didn't change.

They note that some of the paleo dieters complained about the volume of food they had to eat.

This particular version of the paleo diet indeed seems to have potential to help control diabetes in obese type 2's, perhaps even better than an ADA diet, despite a relatively high carbohydrate content. Obviously, it's a very small study and I'd like to see it tested in a larger population for several months, and in type 1 diabetics. But it will be years, if ever, before we see those re-search results. Diabetics alive today have to decide what they'll eat tomorrow.

I wish the researchers had explained why they chose their paleo diet macronutrient breakdown: calorie per-centages from protein, fat, and carbohydrate were 18%, 27%, and 58%, respectively. Perhaps they were trying to match the ratios of the ADA diet. But from what I've read, the average ancestral paleo diet carbo-hydrate energy percentage is 30–35%, not close to 60%. My experience is that reducing carb calorie con-sumption to 30% or less helps even more with glucose control. Reducing carbs that low in this study would have necessitated some drug adjustments and increased the risk of hypoglycemia.

The authors wonder if the high fiber content of the paleo diet drove the lowered glucose levels.

High HDL cholesterol is thought to be protective against coronary artery disease and other types of atherosclerosis. Both diet groups here saw reductions in HDL. That's something to keep an eye on.

The ADA diet group saw a drop in HgbA1c but not fructosamine. I can't explain how HgbA1c goes down over three weeks without a change in fructosamine level.

You have to wonder if the paleo diet results would have been more impressive if the test subjects at baseline had been sicker, with poorly controlled blood pressures and HgbA1c's of 9% or higher. And it sounds like some of these folks would have lost weight if not forced to eat more to keep from losing weight. The Jonsson study (2010) found the paleo diet more satiating than the Mediterranean diet.

ADDITIONAL RESOURCES

John Hawks Weblog
http://johnhawks.net
Paleoanthropology, genetics, and evolution; a massive
database almost equivalent to a paleoanthropology
textbook

John Sorrentino, D.M.D.
http://www.sorrentinodental.com/blog/
Blog of Dr. Sorrentino, a dentist who recommends a
carbohydrate-restricted paleo diet for prevention and
treatment of common dental problems

Diabetes Warrior
http://www.diabetes-warrior.net
Steve Cooksey cured or controls his type 2 diabetes
with the paleo diet

Evolutionary Psychiatry
http://evolutionarypsychiatry.blogspot.com
Blog of psychiatrist Emily Deans, M.D., who is search-
ing for evolutionary solutions to general and mental
health problems

Gnolls.org
http://www.gnolls.org
J. Stanton on reclaiming our evolutionary heritage

Mark's Daily Apple
http://www.marksdailyapple.com
Mark Sisson's website for primal eating (paleo diet plus
dairy); recipes, blog, etc.

Nom Nom Paleo
http://nomnompaleo.com
Pharm.D. Michelle Tam's website; beaucoup recipes

Paleo Infused Nutrition
http://www.paleoinfused.com
Website of Kelly Schmidt, registered dietitian and type 1 diabetic

PaleoHikerMD
http://paleohikermd.com
Website of internist Ernie Garcia, M.D., a paleo diet proponent

Perfect Health Diet
http://perfecthealthdiet.com
Website of paleo-inspired Ph.D.s Paul and Shou-Ching Jaminet; recipes and more

Robb Wolf
http://robbwolf.com
Blog of Robb Wolf, author of *The Paleo Solution*

The Paleo Diet
http://thepaleodiet.com
Website of Loren Cordain, Ph.D.; recipes, blog, paleo diet education

The Poor, Misunderstood Calorie
http://caloriesproper.com
Blog of William Lagakos, Ph.D.; all about energy balance with a focus on food, hormones, weight loss

Rogue Health and Fitness
http://roguehealthandfitness.com
P.D. Mangan's blog on science-based health, fitness, and anti-aging for men

DEFINITIONS OF DIABETES, PREDIABETES, AND GESTATIONAL DIABETES

DIABETES

Guidelines issued by the American Diabetes Association define adult, non-pregnant diabetes thusly:
- Fasting blood sugar 126 mg/dl (7 mmol/l) or greater, or
- Blood sugar 200 mg/dl (11.1 mmol/l) or greater two hours after ingesting 75 grams of glucose (an oral glucose tolerance test), or
- Hemoglobin A1c 6.5% or greater (48 mmol/mol), or
- Random ("casual") blood sugar 200 mg/dl (11.1 mmol/l) or greater, plus symptoms of hyperglycemia (thirst, frequent and voluminous urination, weight loss, blurry vision)

Hemoglobin A1c is an indicator of average blood sugar readings over the prior three months. The average healthy non-diabetic adult hemoglobin A1c is 5% and translates into an average blood sugar of 100 mg/dl (5.6 mmol/l). This will vary a bit from lab to lab. Most healthy non-diabetics would be under 5.7%.

To confirm the diagnosis, always repeat the test on a subsequent day if there are no clear-cut symptoms of hyperglycemia. Yes, sometimes laboratories make mistakes. You don't want to be labeled diabetic or prediabetic if you're not really. A diagnosis of diabetes could raise your premium for health and life insurance. Would prediabetes? Maybe.

PREDIABETES

The ADA also has criteria for diagnosis of prediabetes in non-pregnant adults. There are two forms of prediabetes: impaired fasting glucose and impaired glucose tolerance. Here are the numbers:

- Impaired fasting glucose: fasting blood sugar 100–125 mg/dl (5.6–6.9 mmol/l)
- Impaired glucose tolerance): blood sugar 140–199 mg/dl (7.8–11 mmol/l) two hours after ingesting 75 grams of glucose (an oral glucose tolerance test)
- Hemoglobin A1c in the range of 5.7 to 6.4% (39–46 mmol/mol)

Compared to impaired fasting glucose, impaired glucose tolerance may be a better predictor of increased risk of cardiovascular disease and death. So some researchers and clinicians focus on preventing high blood sugar swings after meals.

GESTATIONAL DIABETES

Gestational diabetes occurs in 5% of pregnancies in the U.S., affecting more than 240,000 births annually. Compared to Caucasians, gestational diabetes mellitus (GDM) occurs more often in Blacks, Native Americans, Asians, and Latinos.

Numerous problems are associated with GDM, for both the mother and the baby:

- dangerously high blood pressure (preeclampsia)
- excessive amount of amniotic fluid (the baby in the uterus floats in this fluid)
- delivery requiring an operation
- early or premature delivery
- death of the baby
- birth trauma, such as broken bones or nerve injury

- metabolic problems in the baby (low blood sugar, for example)
- abnormally large baby (macrosomia, a major problem)

Diabetic ketoacidosis—a life-threatening complication of diabetes—is rare in GDM.

All pregnancies are characterized by some degree of insulin resistance and high insulin levels: they are necessary for the baby. Nevertheless, healthy pregnant women run blood sugars 20% lower than when they're not pregnant.

Most women should undergo a screening test for gestational diabetes around the 24th to 28th week of pregnancy. Screen earlier if undiagnosed type 2 diabetes is suspected or if risk factors for diabetes are present. The American Diabetes Association (2014 guidelines) recommends either one of two screening tests:

1) "One-step test." It's a morning oral glucose tolerance test after at least eight hours of fasting. Fasting blood sugar is tested then the woman drinks 75 grams oral of glucose. Blood sugar is tested again one and two hours later. This blood sample is obtained by a needle in a vein, not by finger prick. Gestational diabetes is diagnosed if any of the following apply: 1) fasting glucose is 92 mg/dl (5.1 mmol/l) or higher, 2) One-hour level is 180 mg/dl (10.0 mmol/l) or higher, or 3) two-hour level is 153 mg/dl (8.5 mmol/l) or higher.

2) "Two-step test." This is a nonfasting test with only one needle-stick. The woman drinks 50 grams of glucose; plasma glucose is tested one hour later. But if it's over 140 mg/dl (10.0 mmol/l), that's a flunk and a three-hour 100-gram oral glucose tolerance test in the fasting state must be done (step two). Gestational diabetes is present if the three-hour glucose is 140 mg/dl (7.8 mmol/l) or higher.

Other experts say the diagnosis requires two or more of the following:
- fasting blood sugar > 95 mg/dl (5.3 mmol/l)
- 1-hour blood sugar > 180 mg/dl (10 mmol/l)
- 2-hour blood sugar > 155 mg/dl (8.6 mmol/l)
- 3-hour blood sugar > 140 mg/dl (7.8 mmol/l)

There's no need for the screening test if a random blood sugar is over 200 mg/dl (11.1 mmol/l) or a fasting sugar is over 126 mg/dl: those numbers already define diabetes, assuming they are confirmed with a second high reading. A random blood sugar over 200 mg/dl (11.1 mmol/l) should be repeated for confirmation. Gestational diabetes can be diagnosed at the first prenatal visit if fasting blood sugar is 92 or over mg/dl (5.1 mmol/l or over) but under 126 mg/dl (7 mmol/l), or if hemoglobin A1c at the first prenatal visit is 6.5% or greater.

Women with diabetes in the first trimester (first three months of pregnancy) have overt diabetes, not gestational diabetes.

Having had gestational diabetes, the mother is at high risk of developing typical non-pregnant diabetes in the future. She should be screened for the development of diabetes and prediabetes at least every three years. Regular exercise and loss of excess weight substantially decrease the odds of developing diabetes.

NEWER THEORIES ON THE CAUSE OF TYPE 2 DIABETES

PORIES AND DOHM: HYPERINSULINEMIA AND THE UNIDENTIFIED DIABETOGENIC SIGNAL

Excessive insulin output by the pancreas (hyperinsulinemia) is the underlying cause of type 2 diabetes, according to a hypothesis from Walter Pories, M.D., and G. Lynis Dohm, Ph.D. The cause of the hyperinsulinemia is a yet-to-be-identified "diabetogenic signal" to the pancreas from the gastrointestinal tract (49).

They base their hypothesis on the well-known cure or remission of many cases of type 2 diabetes quite soon after roux-en-y gastric bypass surgery (RYGB) done for weight loss. (Recent data indicate that six years after surgery, the diabetes has recurred in about a third of cases.) Elevated fasting insulin levels return to normal within a week of RYGB and remain normal for at least three months. Also soon after surgery, the pancreas recovers the ability to respond to a meal with an appropriate insulin spike. Remission or cure of type 2 diabetes after RYGB is independent of changes in weight, insulin sensitivity, or free fatty acids.

Bariatric surgery provides us with a "natural" experiment into the mechanisms behind type 2 diabetes.

The primary anatomic change with RYGB is exclusion of food from a portion of the gastrointestinal tract, which must send a signal to the pancreas resulting in lower insulin levels, according to Pories and Dohm. (RYGB prevents food from hitting most of the stomach and the first part of the small intestine.)

275

Why would fasting blood sugar levels fall so soon after RYGB? To understand, you have to know that fasting glucose levels primarily reflect glucose production by the liver (gluconeogenesis). It's regulated by insulin and other hormones. Insulin generally suppresses gluconeogenesis. The lower insulin levels after surgery should raise fasting glucose levels then, don't you think? But that's not the case.

Pories and Dohm surmise that correction of hyperinsulinemia after surgery leads to fewer glucose building blocks (pyruvate, alanine, and especially lactate) delivered from muscles to the liver for glucose production. Their explanation involves an upregulated Cori cycle, etc. It's pretty difficult to follow and boring unless you're a biochemist.

The theory we're talking about is contrary to the leading theory that insulin resistance causes hyperinsulinemia. Our guys are suggesting it's the other way around: hyperinsulinemia causes insulin resistance. It's a chicken or the egg sort of thing.

If they're right, Pories and Dohm say we need to re-think the idea of treating type 2 diabetes with insulin except in the very late stages when there may be no alternative. (I would add my concern about using insulin secretagogues (e.g., sulfonylureas and meglitinides) in that case also.) If high insulin levels are the culprit, you don't want to augment them, adding fuel to the fire.

We'd also need to figure out what is the identity and source of the "diabetogenic signal" from the gastrointestinal tract to the pancreas that causes hyperinsulinemia. A number of stomach and intestinal hormones can affect insulin production by the pancreas; these were not mentioned specifically by Pories and Dohm. Examples are GIP and GLP-1 (glucose-dependent insulinotropic polypeptide and glucagon-like peptide-1).

ROY TAYLOR: INTRA-ORGAN FAT CAUSES TYPE 2 DIABETES

According to Roy Taylor, M.D., "type 2 diabetes is a potentially reversible metabolic state precipitated by the single cause of chronic excess intra-organ fat." The organs accumulating fat are the pancreas and liver (50). He is certain "...that the disease process can be halted with restoration of normal carbohydrate and fat metabolism."

Do you remember that report in 2011 touting cure of type 2 diabetes with a very low calorie diet? I didn't think so. Taylor was the leader. The study involved only 11 patients, eating 600 calories a day for eight weeks. You're probably eating 1,800 to 3,000 calories daily now, so cutting to 600 is drastic.

Dr. Taylor says that severe calorie restriction is similar to the effect of bariatric surgery in curing or controlling diabetes. Within a week of either intervention, liver fat content is greatly reduced, liver insulin sensitivity returns, and fasting blood sugar levels can return to normal. During the first eight weeks after intervention, pancreatic fat content falls, with associated steadily increasing rates of insulin secretion by the pancreas beta cells.

Here are some scattered points from Dr. Taylor.

- In type 2 diabetes, improvement in fasting blood sugar reflects improved liver insulin sensitivity more than muscle insulin sensitivity.
- The more fat accumulation in the liver, the less it is sensitive to insulin. If a type 2 is treated with insulin, the required insulin dose is positively linked to how much fat is in the liver.

- In a type 2 who starts insulin injections, liver fat stores tend to decrease. That's because of suppression of the body's own insulin delivery from the pancreas to the liver via the portal vein.
- Whether obese or not, those with higher circulating insulin levels "...have markedly increased rates of hepatic de novo lipogenesis." That means their livers are making fat. That fat (triglycerides or triacylglycerol) will be either burned in the liver for energy (oxidized), pushed into the blood stream for use elsewhere, or stored in the liver. Fatty acids are components of triglycerides. Excessive fatty acid intermediaries in liver cells—diglycerides and ceramide—are thought to interfere with insulin's action, i.e., contribute to insulin resistance in the liver.
- "Fasting plasma glucose concentration depends entirely on the fasting rate of hepatic [liver] glucose production and, hence, on its sensitivity to suppression by insulin."
- Physical activity, low-calorie diets, and thiazolidinediones reduce the pancreas' insulin output and reduce liver fat levels.
- Most type 2 diabetics have above-average liver fat content.
- Type 2 diabetics have on average only half of the pancreas beta cell mass of non-diabetics. As the years pass, more beta cells are lost. Is there a way to preserve these insulin-producing cells, or to increase their numbers? "...it is conceivable that removal of adverse factors could result in restoration of normal beta cell number, even late in the disease."
- "Chronic exposure of [pancreatic] beta cells to triacylglycerol [triglycerides] or fatty acids...decreases beta cell capacity to respond to an acute increase in glucose levels." In test tubes, fatty acids inhibit formation of new beta

cells, an effect enhanced by increased glucose concentration.

- There's a fair amount of overlap in pancreas fat content comparing type 2 diabetics and non-diabetics. It may be that people with type 2 diabetes are somehow more susceptible to adverse effects of the fat via genetic and epigenetic factors.

- "If a person has type 2 diabetes, there is more fat in the liver and pancreas than he or she can cope with."

- Here's Dr. Taylor's Twin Cycle Hypothesis of Etiology of Type 2 Diabetes: "The accumulation of fat in liver and secondarily in the pancreas will lead to self-reinforcing cycles that interact to bring about type 2 diabetes. Fatty liver leads to impaired fasting glucose metabolism and increases export of VLDL triacylglcerol [triglycerides], which increases fat delivery to all tissues, including the [pancreas] islets. The liver and pancreas cycles drive onward after diagnosis with steadily decreasing beta cell function. However, of note, observations of the reversal of type 2 diabetes confirm that if the primary influence of positive calorie balance is removed, the processes are reversible."

- "The extent of weight gloss required to reverse type 2 diabetes is much greater than conventionally advised." We're looking at around 15 kg (33 lb) or 20% of body weight, assuming the patient is obese to start. "The initial major loss of body weight demands a substantial reduction in energy intake. After weight loss, steady weight is most effectively achieved by a combination of dietary restriction and physical activity."

Dr. Taylor doesn't specify how much calorie restriction he recommends, but reading between the lines, I think he likes his 600 calories a day for eight weeks program. Kids, do not try this at home! It's dangerous without medical supervision, and difficult to maintain, which is probably good. I suspect a variety of existing ketogenic diets may be just as successful and more realistic, even if it takes more than eight weeks. I wonder how many of the 11 diabetes "cures" from the 2011 study have persisted.

ROGER UNGER: THE GLUCAGON-CENTRIC DIABETES MODEL

Perhaps we've been wrong about diabetes all along: the problem isn't so much with insulin as with glucagon.

At least one diabetes researcher would say that's the case. Roger Unger, M.D., is a professor at the University of Texas Southwestern Medical Center.

Glucagon is a hormone secreted by the alpha cells of the pancreas; it raises blood sugar. (There are also glucagon-secreting alpha cells in the lining of the stomach, and I believe also in the duodenum.) In the pancreas, the insulin-producing beta cells are adjacent to the glucagon-secreting alpha cells. Released insulin directly suppresses glucagon. If insulin doesn't suppress glucagon, your blood sugar goes up. Often that's beneficial, even life-saving. But if your blood sugar's too high, as in diabetes, maybe you've got too much glucagon action rather than too little insulin action.

Dr. Unger says that insulin regulates glucagon. If your sugar's too high, your insulin isn't adequately keeping a lid on glucagon. Without glucagon, your blood sugar wouldn't be high. *Without glucagon, your blood sugar wouldn't be high.* Got it? All known forms of diabetes mellitus have been found to have high glucagon levels (if not in peripheral blood, then in veins draining glucagon-secreting organs).

This is pretty well proven in mice. And maybe hamsters. I don't know if we have all the pertinent evidence in humans, because it's harder to do the testing.

280

Here's Dr. Unger's glucagon-centric theory of the pathway to insulin-resistant type 2 diabetes: First we over-eat too many calories, leading to insulin over-secretion, leading to increased fat production (lipogenesis) and storage in pancreatic islet cells as triglycerides, in turn leading to increased ceramide (which is toxic) in those islet cells, leading to pancreas beta cell death (apoptosis) and insulin resistance in the alpha cell (so glucagon is over-produced), all culminating in type 2 diabetes. If you're like me, you may need to read that last sentence three or four times to get it. It's not easy. Dr. Unger makes it clearer in a YouTube video (51).

If this is all true, so what? It could lead to some new and more effective treatments for diabetes. Dr. Unger says that in type 2 diabetes, we need to suppress glucagon. Potential ways to do that include a chemical called somatostatin, glucagon receptor antibodies, and leptin. The glucagon-centric theory of diabetes also explains why type 1 diabetics rarely have totally normal blood sugars no matter how hard they try: we're ignoring the glucagon side of the equation. I don't yet understand his argument, but he also says that giving higher doses of insulin to type 2 diabetics may well be harmful. I'm guessing the insulin leads to increased accumulation of lipids and the toxic ceramide in cells.

RECIPE INDEX

INDEX

ABOUT THE AUTHORS

Steve Parker, M.D., is an Internal Medicine specialist with three decades' experience treating diabetes and prediabetes. He lives with his wife (Sunny) and children in Scottsdale, Arizona (USA), and practices medicine full-time as a hospitalist. He vows to keep practicing until he gets it right. Dr. Parker's other books include:

The Advanced Mediterranean Diet: Lose Weight, Feel Better, Live Longer (2nd Edition)

Conquer Diabetes and Prediabetes: The Low-Carb Mediterranean Diet

KMD: Ketogenic Mediterranean Diet

Connect with Dr. Parker:

Twitter: @steveparkermd
Blogs:
    Paleo Diabetic
       http://paleodiabetic.com
    Diabetic Mediterranean Diet
       http://diabeticmediterraneandiet.com
    Advanced Mediterranean Life
       http://advancedmediterranean.com
E-mail: steveparkermd@gmail.com. Due to the volume of e-mail he receives, Dr. Parker may not be able to respond to you in a timely fashion, or at all. He cannot provide you with personal medical advice via e-mail.

If you faithfully followed the Paleobetic Diet for several weeks or months, the authors would love to get feedback from you. Did it lower your blood sugars? Did you lose any excess weight? Did you have hypo-glycemic episodes or other adverse effects? Did your blood pressure or lipids (cholesterols and triglycer-ides) change? Were you able to reduce your diabetic drugs? Did you like the recipes? You can reach Dr. Parker via e-mail at steveparkermd@gmail.com. He won't share your personal information with anyone without your consent. Also feel free also to share your experience at various online diabetes forums.

The authors would be much obliged if you left a re-view of the book at Amazon.com and similar venues. They are convinced the Paleobetic Diet is a healthful way of eating. Would you please help them spread the word?

Printed in Poland
by Amazon Fulfillment
Poland Sp. z o.o., Wrocław